Was it something you ate?

Was it something you ate?

Food intolerance: what causes it and how to avoid it

John Emsley and Peter Fell

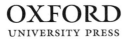

OXFORD
UNIVERSITY PRESS

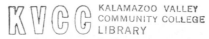

OXFORD
UNIVERSITY PRESS

Great Clarendon Street, Oxford OX2 6DP

Oxford University Press is a department of the University of Oxford.
It furthers the University's objective of excellence in research, scholarship,
and education by publishing worldwide in

Oxford   New York
Athens   Auckland   Bangkok   Bogotá   Buenos Aires   Calcutta
Cape Town   Chennai   Dar es Salaam   Delhi   Florence   Hong Kong   Istanbul
Karachi   Kuala Lumpur   Madrid   Melbourne   Mexico City   Mumbai
Nairobi   Paris   São Paulo   Singapore   Taipei   Tokyo   Toronto   Warsaw

and with associated companies in   Berlin   Ibadan

Oxford is a registered trade mark of Oxford University Press
in the UK and in certain other countries

Published in the United States
by Oxford University Press Inc., New York

© John Emsley and Peter Fell, 1999

A catalogue record for this book is available from the British Library

Library of Congress Cataloging in Publication Data
Emsley, John.
Was it something you ate?: food intolerance, what causes it and
how to avoid it/John Emsley and Peter Fell.
Includes bibliographical references and index.
ISBN 0 19 850443 8 (Hbk)

1. Food–Toxicology.   2. Nutritionally induced diseases.
I. Fell, Peter.   II. Title.
RA 1258.E48 1999   615.9'54–dc21   99-15702

Typeset by Newgen Imaging Systems (P) Ltd., Chennai, India

Printed in Great Britain
on acid-free paper by
Biddles Ltd.,
Guildford & King's Lynn

Contents

Acknowledgements

We would like to thank Mrs V. Fell, Mrs J. Weston, and Mrs H. M. Glyn-Davies for helping with nutritional information, and Dr T. P. Coultate for useful advice on food chemistry.

Introduction

Humans very quickly learn not to eat foods that upset them, and we each have a few that we assiduously avoid, even though we see others enjoying them with impunity. If a young child eats something which makes it sick, then it is very difficult to persuade that child to eat the same food again. The distressing act of vomiting becomes associated with that particular food, and it teaches the child a lesson it may never forget. When we are older we learn that food may poison us for a variety of reasons—it may be contaminated with bacteria or fungi; it may be slightly poisonous and we have eaten too much; or it may contain something to which we really are allergic.

Alcohol is an example of a food that is moderately poisonous, but such is the pleasure derived from drinking it, that we ignore this inconvenient fact, and we suffer the consequences the following day. We understand the risk but have decided to ignore the outcome, and when we groan under a hangover the next morning we know the cause and accept the punishment. It rarely prevents us repeating the experience, even though we know that in the long term it may be endangering our life.

It is when we suffer the consequences without realising their cause, that we may decide that something in our diet has affected us. Often you hear people say, as they refuse a particular food, 'it doesn't agree with me' or 'I like it, but it doesn't like me'—they know they will suffer if they eat it. They may even assert that they are *allergic* to it, although this is unlikely. It is more likely that they are *intolerant* of something it contains, though what that something is they rarely discover.

Intolerance and allergy are very different, so how do you tell one from the other?

An *allergic* response occurs when our body's immune system reacts adversely to even a tiny amount of a particular food (usually some form of protein) or environmental agent (often an animal enzyme, or plant pollen). Allergic reactions are out of all proportion to the amount of alien material we take into our body—indeed, they can sometimes be so severe as to be fatal. This can happen with peanuts.

Intolerance, on the other hand, is caused by the body's inability to detoxify certain components in food. The immune system itself is not involved, and often the response is the same as if the agent were indeed a poison to be disposed of. Intolerance may take two forms: either the component is a non-nutrient to be got rid of as quickly as possible, or it is a nutrient, but our genetic makeup is such that we can not digest it like other people. In the former case our body's response is likely to be related to the amount of the agent we have consumed. In the latter case we lack the necessary enzymes to digest it. Enzymes are needed by the body to carry out the hundreds of chemical reactions that transform one substance into another, and if we lack a particular digestive enzyme we will experience a problem with our food. For example, lactose is present in all milk except soya milk, and the enzyme lactase is needed to digest it. Human babies, in common with all other mammals, produce this enzyme in the small intestine, but once they are weaned they may stop secreting it (this is especially true of oriental people). Another food, gluten, which occurs in wheat, can also present problems for those unable to digest it. When this happens our body copes as best it can, but if we are one of the unlucky few who are so affected we have to learn which foods to avoid. Once the problem is diagnosed, we can adjust our diet accordingly. Any food can cause this sort of intolerance reaction, but the most common are milk, peanuts, eggs, fish, shellfish, and wheat.

To keep our body healthy we need our diet to supply it with energy, plus nutrients that can be used to create new cells and to keep existing ones working properly. Carbohydrates and fats provide mainly energy, although some of these food components are needed to build new tissue. Proteins provide the building blocks for new tissue, but these too can be broken down to release the energy they contain. Vitamins and minerals are essential chemicals that our body needs if it is to operate properly.

Apart from these key components of our food there are other chemicals that our body can not use for energy or nutrition, but which might serve some other useful purpose. For example, cellulose is an indigestible form of carbohydrate which is often referred to as fibre, and while it supplies neither energy nor essential nutrients, it is nevertheless important because it provides bulk for our intestines, to keep them working efficiently, and it can absorb excess body chemicals, such as cholesterol, and carry them out of the system.

Finally, there are the other non-nutrients—they are what this book is all about. These non-nutrients may occur naturally in our food, such as biogenic amines, or be deliberate or accidental contaminants from food processing. Some, such as sulfites, are added to protect food against contamination by preventing the growth of undesirable microorganisms; others, such as monosodium glutamate, are used to enhance the taste; while a few are deliberately taken, such as caffeine, because of the effect they have on us. The table lists some of the more common ones. In moderation, none of these non-nutrients threatens us, but we can eat meals where a combination of foods can deliver such a large dose of one of them that it provokes a toxic response—an intolerance reaction—from our body. Our defences swing into action, and we suffer the consequences.

For example, monosodium glutamate (MSG) caused one of the major food scares of recent years. Reports like the one opposite explain why this flavour-enhancing chemical became so unpopular in the 1980s and early 1990s.

This British tabloid newspaper's account is exaggerating what it reports: MSG does not cause paralysis. Much more likely are other symptoms, such as flushing, and pins and needles. The cause of the diners' food intolerance reaction was almost certainly the Chinese meal, and the crab soup was no doubt heavily laced with MSG. Rarely does MSG, which is a perfectly natural component of many foods, cause such severe symptoms because we

Some common non-nutrients that are in everyday foods.

Non-nutrient	Description	Found in
Aflatoxin	natural toxin, produced by moulds	cow's milk, egg white, corn, peanuts, Brazil, nuts, etc.
Benzoic acid	natural chemical, also used as a preservative	some berries; synthetic version added to pizzas, yoghurts, fruit drinks, etc.
Caffeine,	stimulant	coffee, tea, colas, cocoa powder, etc.
Erythrosine BS	colouring agent	canned fruit, salami, sausages, cake decorations, marshmallow, etc.
Monosodium glutamate (MSG)	flavour enhancer	processed savoury foods and snacks, Camembert cheese, fish fingers, packet soups, etc.
Octopamine	natural amine	ham, cows milk, pork, mutton, lobster
Phenylethylamine	natural amine	chocolate and chocolate products
Potassium nitrite	preservative	sausages, hot dogs, salami, bacon, pâté, Edam cheese, pizzas, etc.
Saccharin	artificial sweetener	diet drinks and processed foods
Sulfites, metabisulfites	antioxidants, preservatives	dried fruits, mincemeat, pickles, instant soups, instant mashed potato, milk shake syrup, fruit juices and drinks
Solanine	natural toxin	tomato, potato, green and coloured peppers, chillies, aubergine/eggplant, black pepper, etc.
Sorbic acid	natural antifungal agent and preservative	toppings, soup concentrates, yoghurt, cakes, soft drinks, red wine, etc.
Sunset yellow FCF	colouring agent	fruit drink concentrates, yoghurts, marzipan, packet pudding mixes, etc.
Tartrazine	colouring agent	quick-set gels, manufactured bread crumbs, cheese sauce mixes, soft drinks
Tyramine	natural amine	spinach, banana, tomato, potato, pork, chicken, cows' milk

rarely consume too much at any one meal. Chapter 1 offers a closer look at this highly controversial food component.

In the last 20 years many books have been written warning of supposed dangers in our food. Some of these books grossly exaggerate the effects of substances such as traces of the pesticides used in farming, or the additives used in food processing. There was little scientific backing for the claims being made, which were often little more than alarmist speculation. Nevertheless, people changed their eating habits to avoid these supposedly dangerous chemicals, often at great expense, both financial and emotional. Those who believed these messages of alarm began to see food not as something to be enjoyed, but as a hidden threat to their health. Rarely did the advice help the reader to understand what was going on, because there was little science in what was being said. In *Was it something you ate?* we offer no advice that is not medically or scientifically substantiated. Here, in straightforward language, is an explanation of how certain chemicals can affect us, how we can discover those we are particularly sensitive to, and what we can do to avoid getting an excess of them at any one time.

There can be dangers lurking in food that will make anyone ill who eats it. Such dangers are generally caused by microbes, which may be bacteria, fungi, yeasts, moulds, or viruses, but such food poisoning can be prevented by the kind of simple hygiene that even our grandparents were aware of: cooking food thoroughly to destroy bacteria; storing food in a refrigerator to prevent moulds multiplying; keeping kitchen surfaces clean; washing hands before preparing meals; and disinfecting cloths that are used in the kitchen.

But even when you have taken all these precautions, you may still suffer a bad reaction from a meal. Then it is time to think about what you have eaten, and the natural tendency is to single out something unusual about the meal, such as a new type of cheese or wine, and blame your sickness on that. Of course, you may be right in your suspicions: that particular food may be the cause because it delivered a dose of an unwanted non-nutrient that your body responded to adversely. Alternatively, the whole meal may have provided an accumulation of small doses of this non-nutrient that collectively amounted to more than your body could eliminate.

How then do we safeguard ourselves against this happening? First, we need to know what the likely non-nutrients are that can make us ill, and then we need to know how to avoid an overload of whichever affects us. We can not guarantee that *Was it something you ate?* will uncover your particular problem, but there is a good chance that it will.

This is not another book that promises a remarkable new diet that will ensure that you live to a ripe old age, and avoid heart disease and cancer. That is not our purpose, although we end the book with a chapter of advice that we think might give you a better quality of life, and a healthy old age. Our main objective is to help you get more enjoyment out of life by taking away some of the mystery surrounding food intolerance. Understand the role of a few simple chemicals—some that are natural, and some that are added with good intentions—and you will be in a better position to avoid those that trigger your body's detoxification defences.

CHAPTER 1

Monosodium glutamate

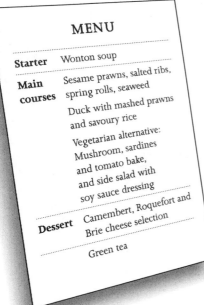

MENU

Starter Wonton soup

Main courses Sesame prawns, salted ribs, spring rolls, seaweed

Duck with mashed prawns and savoury rice

Vegetarian alternative: Mushroom, sardines and tomato bake, and side salad with soy sauce dressing

Dessert Camembert, Roquefort and Brie cheese selection

Green tea

If you ate the above meal you might well suffer some discomfort afterwards, because you would almost certainly have consumed more than 3 grams of monosodium glutamate (MSG), which is commonly used as a flavour enhancer, particularly in oriental cooking. For some people this would be enough to trigger an intolerance reaction of dry mouth, hot cheeks, itchy neck, and a headache—in other words the infamous Chinese Restaurant Syndrome (CRS). But if you are particularly sensitive to MSG you don't need to eat in such a place to suffer from CRS, as the case study in the box shows.

Case study: **Bingo!**

Rory was a 32-year-old New Zealander who arrived in the UK with his new wife. They planned to work for a few months to earn enough money to buy a camping van, and then tour Europe. He soon found a job as a computer systems adviser, but this entailed living most of the week away from home, which meant a complete change of diet from the home cooking he had been used to. Rory was a keen sportsman and kept fit by always going for a work-out immediately after his day's work and before taking his evening meal.

A few weeks into the job found him suffering migraines, headaches, nausea, and nightmares, sometimes so vivid that he could not get back to sleep after them. At weekends he would return to his wife and the symptoms would disappear. Then one weekend they went out with friends for a Chinese meal, after which he had an attack far worse than any he had had so far, and he sought medical help. He was referred to a specialist in diet-related disorders.

Rory was advised that the probable cause was MSG, and he was given lists of foods to avoid. As a result he had no further attacks for a while, but then they started again when he stayed at a certain boarding house. He had already explained to the landlady, Mrs Smith, that he must avoid MSG, and she followed his instructions. Yet on three separate occasions the symptoms recurred. When an attack began, after an evening meal of fish, he went to confront her, only to find that Mrs Smith had gone out for the evening to play bingo.

The following morning, she assured him that she was doing what he wished, and that she had used nothing that contained MSG. A week or so later he had another attack, and the week after that, and on both occasions it was on an evening when Mrs Smith was at bingo, leaving her husband to do the cooking for her lodgers.

The following week on bingo night Rory went out for a meal of fish and chips and was unaffected. Later that evening when the couple had gone to bed Rory went down to the kitchen and in the waste bin he found what he had suspected: the wrapper for a cook-in sauce which he knew contained a lot of MSG. Lacking his wife's skill at making meals Mr Smith simply took the easy option on bingo evening, and Rory suffered as a result.

So what is monosodium glutamate? And why should it provoke such a reaction? We might expect this to happen if it were an alien chemical being added to food, but the glutamate of MSG is present naturally in many foods, such as tomatoes and cheese, and our own body makes it, because it is essential to the working of our brain. This is the paradox that needs to be resolved to explain the effect of this common food ingredient.

MSG is the sodium salt of a naturally occurring amino acid, glutamic acid. There are other salts, such as monopotassium glutamate and calcium glutamate, which are also used as flavour enhancers, especially for those who are on a low-sodium diet. The sodium, potassium, and calcium contribute a little to our daily intake of these minerals, but they are not the active part of MSG. The glutamate is the reason why this flavour enhancer is popular: this is the active ingredient.

We can not be *allergic* to MSG because we need glutamate if every cell in our body is to function properly. Some glutamate we make ourselves, some we take from the microbes which live in our gut, and some we absorb from the food we eat. It is this last supply that can cause us to react badly. Glutamate comes in two forms: free glutamate and bound glutamate. Free glutamate, as its name implies, is instantly available to the body, whereas bound glutamate is not, because it is part of the protein component of our food. Bound glutamate only becomes free glutamate as protein is digested by protease enzymes in our gut, which slowly break it down into its component amino acids, of which glutamic acid is but one. Glutamate released from protein can not provide the *instant* excess that too much MSG can produce.

Table 1.1 shows the two kinds of glutamate in a selection of foods, arranged in order of the amount of free glutamate. We could have headed the list with the edible seaweed called

Table 1.1 MSG in foods (quantities are milligrams of MSG per 100 g of food).

Food	Free glutamate	Bound glutamate
Parmesan cheese	1200	9800
Peas	200	5600
Tomatoes	140	240
Corn	130	1800
Potatoes	100	270
Spinach	40	290
Chicken	45	3300
Carrots	35	200
Beef	35	2800
Mackerel	35	2400
Pork	25	2300
Eggs	25	1600
Onions	20	210
Lamb	20	2700
Salmon	20	2200
Cod	10	2100

kelp, which has 2240 mg of free glutamate per 100 g (which is 2.24% by weight), but this is not usually eaten as a food in the West.

It is free glutamate that causes the discomfort of a toxic reaction if we are the one person in a thousand or so whose detoxifying capability can not cope with a sudden overload. This is most likely to occur when a lot of MSG has been added as a flavour enhancer, a common practice in many Chinese restaurants. Unfortunate diners may then experience the symptoms of the Chinese Restaurant Syndrome.

Chinese restaurant syndrome (CRS)

No Chinese chef worth his salt would cook a meal without using MSG or an ingredient such as soya sauce which is rich in it. Yet it is not only oriental cooking that can be loaded with MSG. This flavour enhancer found its way into processed foods in the West in the 1950s, and in the USA the National Restaurant Association encouraged its use, endorsing it as perfectly safe. In fact, MSG was thought to be so safe that it was not necessary for manufacturers to indicate the amounts that were being added to foods. Some children's snacks contained very high levels, and it was noted that these were particularly attractive to certain children who would tend to eat them to excess. Because of the importance of glutamate as a transmitter of brain signals it was even suggested that this was a good thing, and that it might improve the IQ of mentally retarded children.

For a time in the 1950s and 1960s MSG was even added to infant and formula feeds. This seemed a reasonable thing to do, because the level of glutamate in human breast milk is quite high (22 mg per l00 ml), whereas in cows' milk it is quite low (2 mg per 100 ml). This was stopped when it was thought that MSG might be linked to possible brain damage, although the link was never proved. Nevertheless, the use of MSG was still seen as a good thing in food for children because it would wean them off sugary treats and on to savoury snacks, which were viewed as healthier alternatives.

The general public became aware of CRS in 1968 as a result of the publicity given to a letter in the *New England Journal of Medicine*. This was from Dr Robert Ho Man Kwok, who said he suffered a series of inexplicable symptoms each time he ate at a Chinese restaurant. These began to appear about 20 minutes after he had finished eating, and consisted of his mouth becoming numb, a tingling sensation around his neck, and a delayed-onset headache which started about six hours later. This would last for up to 24 hours, during which time he suffered a prolonged thirst. What was the cause?

A spate of letters followed, from people who had experienced the same effect after eating Chinese food. Other medical journals, such as the *Lancet* and the *British Medical Journal*, reported variants of the condition, and offered suggestions as to its cause. Some sufferers reported chest pains, while others had different types of headaches, and eventually the full set of these food-related symptoms included heart palpitations, dizziness, muscle tightening, nausea, weakness of the upper arms, and pains in the neck. Whatever the combination of these symptoms, they became known as CRS or Kwok's disease. The media took up the story, and soon this hitherto unknown condition began to break out everywhere. Some of its victims were clearly genuine, and their symptoms very real.

Part of the trouble stemmed from the Western approach to eating oriental food. Despite the saltiness and spicy nature of Chinese dishes, Americans in the 1960s were not accustomed to drinking large quantities of liquid with their meals, whereas in Eastern countries, a meal is accompanied with lots of liquid refreshment such wine, beer, and especially tea (although green tea itself contains a little glutamate). Today diners in a Chinese restaurant in the West are also likely to take lots of drink in the form of mineral waters and beers, and the meal should likewise end with copious quantities of green leaf tea. However, thirst was not the only symptom of CRS, and while drinking would help alleviate the condition, it was not a preventative, nor a cure.

Clearly Chinese cooks were to blame, and the villain of the piece was eventually fingered. It was the chemical MSG, which they often used in excess. Most people had never heard of MSG, although the Chinese and Japanese had been using MSG in various forms for centuries. They had been doing so without apparently noticing a restaurant syndrome associated with it, so what was going on?

In 1969 Herbert Schaumburg, of the Albert Einstein College of Medicine in the Bronx, also suffered from CRS and he speculated in the *New England Journal of Medicine* on what the cause might be. He thought it unlikely to be soya sauce or MSG because his family were heavy users of these at home. Nevertheless, within a year he had changed his mind, and he published a paper entitled 'Monosodium glutamate: its pharmacology and role in the Chinese Restaurant Syndrome' in the influential journal *Science*. Schaumburg identified MSG as the causative agent of CRS. The media reported his findings, and spread the simplistic message: avoid MSG and you won't go down with CRS.

So began a food scare that was to last more than 20 years. Some food manufacturers eventually felt obliged to stress on labels that their products contained no MSG. In the USA there was even an activist group, called NOMSG, dedicated to banning the substance. Undoubtedly some people will react badly to a sudden excess of free glutamate in their diet, as we saw in the case study, but they are few and far between. Most people are unaffected by MSG, and, indeed, their body uses it in the same way as it uses the bound glutamate released from proteins.

Glutamate is used by Japanese and Chinese cooks as a flavour enhancer because it has a stimulatory effect on nerve endings—especially those of the mouth and taste buds. The addition of MSG to meat dishes makes them taste meatier, and fish dishes taste more fish-like. In fact MSG will enhance the flavour of any protein food such as meat, fish, shellfish or cheese, making a little of these go a long way. Many traditional dishes combine a small amount of protein with a food high in free glutamate, resulting in a much tastier meal than if the two foods had been cooked or eaten separately. Typical examples of such dishes are to be found not only in China (e.g. pork and prawns) and Japan (fish and seaweed), but also in Italy (cheese and tomato pizza) and France (champignons à la Grecque—marinated mushrooms with fried shallots, tomatoes, tomato puree and herbs—and Camembert cheese). Wherever such dishes are enjoyed around the world, the chances are that they will be too rich in glutamate for some people.

As food ripens it tastes much better, and in a few cases, such as tomatoes, this is due to the formation of high levels of glutamate. This is why tomatoes make an ideal ingredient for so many dishes. Alternatively we can use stock to enhance flavour, and a stock pot has been a traditional part of the French kitchen. This too provides the glutamate for bringing out the flavour of other dishes. Stock is made by simmering meat or fish scraps with vegetables for long periods, which releases glutamate, but most people find it more convenient to use a stock cube. Both the traditional stock pot and the modern stock cube rely on free glutamate to make tasty dishes.

The forgotten fifth flavour

In the West we recognise four basic flavours: sweet, sour, salt, and bitter. These were first identified by the German psychologist Hans Hening in 1916. On the other hand, Chinese cooks work on the principle that there are five basic tastes (sweet, sour, salt, bitter, and hot) supplemented by two others called xiang and xian. Xiang is pungent and aromatic, and is associated with garlic, spring onions, and certain spices, while xian is savoury, and traditionally linked to oyster sauce, shrimp sauce, chicken stock, and meat stock. Xian can be added to a dish by using a dash of soya sauce, or a pinch of MSG.

The concept of a fifth basic taste is now being accepted in the West, and there is good scientific evidence for it. The name being given to the fifth taste is the Japanese word 'umami.' The nearest words in English for describing the flavour sensation of umami are 'meaty' or 'savoury'. We all know foods that taste umami such as Parmesan cheese, lasagne, bouillon, tomato juice, sardines, mackerel, and tuna.

The Japanese have many more umami foods, such as seaweed, green tea, bonito (striped tunny), sea bream, and dried shiitake and matsutake mushrooms. Cooks there are particularly fond of kelp, whose botanical name is *Laminaria japonica*, which is found in cold ocean waters, and which they use to prepare stock for soups. Kelp has particularly high levels of free glutamate.

Umami was only properly recognised as a basic taste early this century. Professor Kikunae Ikeda of the chemistry department of Tokyo Imperial University observed one day that the taste of the tofu (soya-bean curd) he was eating was made doubly delicious when he took a spoonful of kelp broth at the same time. He investigated the broth and isolated from it an acid which he called umami, and which we now know as glutamic acid. He announced his discovery at the 8th International Conference of Applied Chemistry in Washington DC in 1912. In fact glutamic acid had first been isolated by the German scientist Karl Ritthausen in 1866, and he had obtained it from wheat protein or gluten, hence its name.

Today umami is accepted as a basic flavour in its own right. Numerous experiments have failed to create this taste from combinations of sweet, sour, salty, and bitter. More important has been the discovery of specific umami receptor sites in animal taste cells that recognise this flavour. Umami works best in conjunction with salty and sour tastes, rather than with sweet and bitter tastes.

The umami effect arises from three chemicals: monosodium glutamate (MSG), disodium inosinate (DSI), and disodium guanylate (DSG). MSG is the most important in creating the umami effect. In the European system, of giving an E-code number to all approved food additives, MSG is E621. DSI is second in importance, and this is particularly abundant in sardines, bonito, mackerel, tuna, and pork. DSI is still waiting E-code status, although it has already been given the number 631. The third umami component is DSG, recognised only in 1960 by Dr Akira Kuninaka. This is most common in mushrooms such as shiitake, matsutake, enokitake, and truffle. The combination of DSI and DSG has the code number 635.

The umami flavour chemicals are dependent on one another for maximum effect. When MSG and DSI come together they enhance umami much more than the simple combination would lead us to expect. A chemical reaction occurs between them to produce a umami response that is eight times stronger than that produced by either chemical on its own. When Italian cooks put tomatoes and cheese on a pizza they bring together MSG and DSI and produce a umami-type flavour. Sprinkling Parmesan cheese on to minestrone soup does the same. In Japan, combining seaweed and bonito brings MSG and DSI together to make a stock for soups. And when we add a dash of soya sauce, a spoonful of gravy granules, or a stock cube (even a vegetarian one) to our cooking we are doing exactly the same.

If you choose to cook with MSG then the recommended amounts are as follows (for dishes designed for four people):

- **soups:** up to half a teaspoon (5 g) depending on the soup;
- **fried noodles or fried rice:** one level teaspoon (10 g);
- **meat and fish dishes:** half a teaspoon (5 g).

Clearly a meal in a Chinese restaurant with all these dishes would provide each person with 5 grams, which is more than enough to trigger Kwok's disease in anyone who was intolerant of high doses of free glutamate.

If you buy convenience foods, the MSG will have already been added. Those that are particularly rich in this flavour enhancer are frozen dinners, savoury snacks, spice mixes, canned and packet soups, cook-in sauces, savoury sauces, sausages, and hams. If you suspect that you are intolerant of high levels of glutamate these are the foods to avoid, but bear in mind there are many natural sources of free glutamate, as Table 1.1 shows.

The chemistry and biology of MSG and glutamate

Protein is made of amino acids, of which glutamic acid is one of the most abundant—it sometimes accounts for 20% of protein. Some foods are even higher in glutamate, such as milk proteins, which contain 22%, and wheat protein (31%). Our muscles and many other organs are made up of amino acids linked one to the other in long chains. There are 20 different kinds, some of which we can make in our body. Those we can not make for ourselves must come from our diet, and these are referred to as *essential* amino acids. Glutamate is not one of these, because cells can produce it for themselves. We need glutamate because several other amino acids are made from it in our body, but perhaps its most important function is to act as a neurotransmitter in the brain, carrying nerve impulses from one neuron to the next. Brain cells actually manufacture their own supply of glutamate because it can not pass through the barrier that protects the brain, and which allows only essential components in the bloodstream to pass directly into the brain.

MSG is manufactured industrially from molasses, which is a by-product of sugar cane or sugar beet refining. Molasses is rich in glucose, and this can be turned into glutamic acid by fermenting it with a culture called *Coynebacterium helassecola* in the presence of ammonia gas. The glutamic acid that forms is first purified by crystallisation, and then the crystals are redissolved in fresh water and the acid neutralised to form the sodium salt. The solution is then decolorised and its volume reduced until pure white crystals of MSG grow from it. These are dried, packed, and shipped. The crystals are rather like table salt, and MSG is easy to store and use in this form. As in all salts there is only a loose association between the sodium and the glutamate, and when MSG is dissolved in water, or present in foods and in the body, the sodium breaks away, leaving the free glutamate.

In the acidic conditions of the stomach, MSG will revert to glutamic acid itself, and so is exactly the same as the glutamic acid that is released when a food protein is broken down by digestive enzymes. Chemically there is nothing to distinguish the glutamic acid of digested protein from that of MSG. The body can absorb both equally well through the intestine wall. Soon after it is absorbed, glutamic acid undergoes a transformation, loosing one of its acid groups and a carbon, to become the simpler amino acid, alanine. This is then delivered all round the body wherever new tissue is being made or energy is required.

The average person gets about 10 g of bound glutamate and about 1 g of free glutamate from their food every day, and about 0.5 g of added MSG. At the same time the body makes 50 g of glutamate for its own use. While this may appear to make the intake of MSG from processed food seem rather trivial, we should bear in mind that 0.5 g is for a typical person, and some people may take in much larger amounts, especially if they are attracted to oriental foods and savoury snacks. The average person weighing 70 kg contains 1800 g of glutamate in their body, almost all bound up as protein, but around 10 g is there as free glutamate. The free glutamate is mainly in the muscles (6 g) and brain (2.5 g), with the rest in the liver, kidneys, and a little in the blood. Our body produces it from the break-down of body protein, from other amino acids which it can convert to glutamate, and it can even make some from glucose.

We excrete glutamate from our body to the extent of around 16 g per day in faeces and urine, and by loss of skin.

When glutamate gets out of control

Strokes are the third-largest cause of death in the West, after cancer and heart disease. What used to be puzzling about a stroke, and other types of severe head injury, was the slow pattern of brain damage which only begins to be noticeable after a few days, but then becomes progressively worse. The victim also becomes aware that this is occuring while he or she may be recovering from the original attack. We now know that this damage is caused by the release of glutamate that is produced in the brain.

Glutamate is normally released from brain cells only in the tiny amounts required for mental activity. A stroke interferes with the supply of blood to the brain, and cuts off the essential supplies of oxygen and glucose that the brain must have to supply the energy it needs. Without this energy the brain cells can not control their glutamate reserve, and this begins to leak out of the damaged cells. The glutamate then targets receptors on neighbouring cells, stimulating these continuously until they are literally excited to death. As they die they too release more glutamate and begin to damage their neighbours, and so it goes on.

There are four types of glutamate receptor, one of which is particularly important. Pharmaceutical companies are now bringing out drugs that will block this receptor and protect the brain from the glutamate onslaught. Nature already produces molecules that do this, and the American Garden Spider injects glutamate blockers to paralyse its prey. The spider toxin, called argiotoxin-636, inactivates the glutamate receptors on the nerve cells, denying glutamate molecules access to them. Hunter Jackson and colleagues, of Natural Product Science Inc. of Salt Lake City, tested this toxin on cats that had suffered seizures and they showed it to work as a glutamate-blocker.

Glutamate sensitivity

For most people MSG poses no problem, but for asthmatics and allergy patients an excess of it can cause asthma and upper-airway problems of blocking, sneezing, and running nose. Children with behavioural problems such as hyperactivity and attention deficit can be tested to see if they are intolerant of high doses of glutamate, and if they are they can benefit if MSG is eliminated from their diet. They are tested by being 'challenged' with the component that is suspected of causing the observed symptoms. The offending item is first eliminated from their diet as far as is possible, but is subsequently reintroduced. In the case of MSG, it is reintroduced in tomato juice.

Fatigue is another side-effect of too much MSG. There is a time lag of 12 hours, which makes it difficult for the sufferer to link cause and effect. Glutamate affects the secretion of insulin by the pancreas, and insulin is needed to release the energy we need from the glucose in our cells.

Although free glutamate is natural, the body still has to deal with it when it is confronted with too much at once. It detoxifies the excess glutamate by several mechanisms, the most important of which is via the gut which uses glutamate for 30% of its own energy needs. Here glutamate undergoes a process called deamination, which is removal of the amino part as ammonia. Other systems which remove glutamate are the liver and kidneys where the ammonia released from it can be transferred to another molecule and used there. The enzyme in the body that carries out this process is glutamate dehydrogenase.

These various mechanisms for dealing with too much glutamate can not be speeded up to meet a sudden excess, so there can be an accumulation of glutamate in certain tissues. While the authorities set a safety dose of 10 g of added MSG in the daily diet, this can not take into account the many additional natural sources of glutamate in lots of the things we eat, nor individual sensitivity to excess of this chemical. For some people, an amount greater than 3 g at one time may cause intolerance symptoms, and we can exceed the safe level if we eat lots of foods rich in glutamate, such as the menu given at the start of the chapter. Even so, the adverse effects of excess glutamate depend on the health of the consumer. Healthy people are in no danger. At the end of this chapter there are suggestions for those who suspect they are sensitive to excess free glutamate.

The free glutamate content of foods

MSG is widely used in soups. Packet or canned soups may provide as much as 1.5 g per serving, and wonton soup can deliver three times this amount. Because it is regarded as a safe additive, MSG does not always have to be recorded on the contents label of foods that contain it. Normally, processed foods using MSG would contain less than 0.1 g per 100 g, and with such levels they are completely harmless, but some contain too much. Instant noodles not only have added MSG, but the vegetable and meat extracts they contain may in themselves be rich in free glutamate, perhaps as much as 1.5 g per 100 g.

The use of MSG and other glutamates in foods was reviewed by the Federation of the American Society for Experimental Biology (FASEB), and its 1995 report found no evidence linking MSG to any serious medical problem in the general population. It did find that some people were susceptible to large doses of MSG, and they could develop CRS-type symptoms. At lower levels of consumption, the report said, there was no evidence of anyone being affected; and it recommended to the US Food and Drug Administration (FDA) that MSG be considered a suitable food additive. The FDA's 1993 proposal had required foods with added free glutamate to be labelled 'contains glutamate' even when this was coming from naturally occurring free glutamate. In future, only foods with significant amounts of gluta-mate will need to be labelled.

The other leading organisation, the European Communities' Scientific Committee for Food, declined to set a figure for the Acceptable Daily Intake of MSG, and gave it a 'not speci-fied' classification which is the most favourable grade. The Joint Expert Committee on Food Additives, which is an advisory body of both the Food and Agriculture Organisation and the World Health Organisation of the UN, does not specify an upper safe limit for glutamate, although they caution against adding it to baby feeds.

Table 1.2 gives the amounts of added MSG in some common foods. None of these amounts looks alarmingly high, and in one sitting we are unlikely to exceed the 3 g that can provoke an intolerance reaction. To do this with beef sausages, say, we would need to eat 350 g (12 ounces) which may be perfectly easy to do, but would be most unlikely to happen unless we were addicted to them. Which brings us to the issue we will also deal with in other parts of this book: the unbalanced diet. There is a growing tendency for people to eat the

Table 1.2 Foods with added MSG and the weekly intake of the average person.

Food group	Average free glutamate (%)	Average consumption of this food per week (g)	Calculated intake of free glutamate per week (g)
Fruit and vegetables			
Canned beans	0.14	126	0.18
Canned mushrooms	0.24	36	0.09
Meat and Fish			
Bacon and ham	0.23	26	0.06
Canned ham	0.83	32	0.27
Corned beef	0.41	37	0.15
Sausages (pork)	0.20	38	0.08
Sausages (beef)	0.54	46	0.25
Meat pies	0.10	14	0.01
Burgers	0.56	26	0.15
Lasagne	0.10	158	0.16
Cereals and snacks			
Pizza	0.27	250	0.68
Savoury biscuits/ crackers	0.20	105	0.21
Canned pasta	0.18	35	0.06
Potato crisps/chips	0.91	27	0.26
Miscellaneous			
Nuts	0.48	12	0.06
Cooking sauces	2.06	10	0.21
Canned soups	0.33	77	0.25
Packet soups	3.78	5	0.17
Meat or yeast extracts	8.70	5	0.42
Pickles and sauces	0.60	60	0.37

same kinds of meals day after day, and they tend to be most attracted to those food with high levels of free glutamate and MSG.

The sector of the population that is most at risk of sticking to one kind of food is the 15–25-year-olds who are beyond the stage of being persuaded to eat sensibly by their parents, and who enjoy the freedom to eat a few preferred foods to an unhealthy excess. For most of them, this phase has little effect on their health, and they grow out of the habit or grow bored with the restricted choice they have imposed on themselves. However, they can take in much larger amounts of free glutamate that the rest of the population. Table 1.3 lists a few foods you should be aware of if you are part of this group.

Table 1.3 Too much of a good thing.

Food preferences	Total weekly intake of glutamate for extreme consumers (g)
Potato snacks	13
Cereals	14
Nuts	12
Pizzas and canned pastas	12
Canned soups	13
Packet soups	14

For example, where the average person will eat one packet of potato crisps (known as potato chips in the USA) a day, the 15–25-year-olds often eat three packets a day, totalling around 7 g of free glutamate. Some people even eat these treats at double this rate. The same is true of pizzas, of which the average person eats about 250 g (8 ounces) a week, taking in 0.7 g of free glutamate, but some young people eat more than this each day, and those who like this food often consume around 350 g (12 ounces) per day, taking in more than 8 g of free glutamate a week. Others consume pizzas in excess of this, and if they have a low glutamate intolerance then they might well suffer the symptoms of CRS.

The strange disappearance of CRS

Almost from the start of the Chinese Restaurant Syndrome scare, there were scientists who challenged the theory that MSG was to blame. In 1970 a paper in *Science* reported that humans who had been eating more than 20 g of glutamate a day for many years showed no ill effects. In 1978, in a compilation of scientific papers in the book *Glutamic Acid*, it was stated by one group of toxicologists that they were unable to produce glutamate overdoses in several different species, no matter how much of this chemical was added to their diet. Other reports showed that CRS was ten times more common among those who had heard about it, compared to those who were unaware of the condition. Clearly there was a strong psychosomatic component to this illness, which we now realise would invalidate any epidemiological survey carried out to assess the links between glutamate and CRS.

One of the first to challenge the MSG theory was Richard Kenney of the George Washington University in the USA. In 1986, in the journal *Food Chemistry and Toxicology*, he published findings based on groups of people who suffered from the syndrome and who had volunteered to come forward for testing. All were checked to ensure that they had no biochemical abnormality that could affect their glutamate metabolism. They then took part in double-blind tests with soft drinks, to which either MSG or a placebo had been added. In this type of test, not only does the volunteer not know whether the drink he or she is being given contains the suspected material, but neither does the person carrying out the test. This eliminates any bias or clues that the tester might inadvertently be giving out. The samples are made up independently and then coded so that no-one involved with actual testing knows which samples are which.

When the results of Kenney's test were analysed, they revealed that most of the volunteers suffered psychosomatic symptoms. Often those who drank the placebo went down with a full attack of CRS, while some who drank the concoction laced with MSG were unaffected by it.

Between 1968 and 1990 there were 19 studies carried out to test the impact of MSG on people: about half of these reinforced the link between MSG and CRS, while the others refuted it. The most convincing tests were carried out by Leonid Tarasoff and Michael Kelly of the University of Western Sydney in 1993, and were reported in the journal *Food and Chemical Toxicology*. They looked again at the earlier tests and found that in all of them the people being tested knew that the test was specifically designed to determine the effects of MSG. In some of the tests MSG was even given as a powder to those being tested, and it was thought that this could perhaps be detected by its slight flavour.

Tarasoff and Kelly decided that in their experiments the people who volunteered would not be told what they were testing, but they would be given capsules as part of a study to evaluate a new soft drink. At no stage was MSG mentioned. Again it was a double-blind test of 71 volunteers, some of whom were asked to take capsules that contained either 1.5 or 3 g of MSG, while others took a capsule containing a placebo. Eleven of the volunteers reported some reaction after swallowing the MSG capsules, while 10 reported similar effects from the placebo. The remaining 50 reported no reaction at all. According to Tarasoff and Kelly, MSG was really a scapegoat, and the real villain of CRS is more likely to be some other component, perhaps histamine, which forms during the fermentation of ingredients that are commonly used in Chinese cooking, such as soy sauce, black beans, and shrimp paste. We shall be looking at histamine as a prime cause of food intolerance in Chapter 4.

Dietary advice

If you are one of those people who suspect they suffer some symptoms after eating a high-glutamate meal, then you can test this simply by altering your diet to exclude foods with high levels of MSG or free glutamate. This is fairly easy to do by using the guidelines in the diet chart below. If, after a month, your symptoms have abated or disappeared then you might well consider changing your eating habits permanently to exclude some of the high glutamate foods that you previously enjoyed. (Before you take this step you might check whether MSG really is the problem by 'challenging' your body with a food that is rich in free glutamate, such as tomato juice, to see if the symptoms reappear.)

Examine food labels for lists of ingredients, and look especially for numbers 620–625 (E620–E625 in Europe). Check carefully, because MSG may not be listed under ingredients—it may be listed as a condiment. Eating out may pose a problem because MSG may be added to dishes, or it may be present in one of the ingredients, such as stock. You could

Use this chart if you think you might be intolerant of high levels of free glutamate.

Foods that are low in free glutamate	Foods that are high in free glutamate
Fruit and vegetables	
Apples, pears, oranges, bananas, melons, berries	Grapes, plums, raisins, dried apricots, prunes
Potatoes, carrots, cabbage, beans (all kinds), lettuce, cauliflower, beetroot, swedes, turnip, courgettes/zucchini, cucumber, spinach	Tomatoes, mushrooms, peas, sweetcorn
Meat and fish	
Fresh and freshly prepared foods such as red meat, chicken and fish	
Dairy products	
Eggs, milk (fresh, canned, skimmed, evaporated, condensed, powdered), cream, butter	Cheeses: Roquefort, Parmesan, Gruyère, Gouda, Camembert, Brie
Ice cream, custards, yoghurts	
Cheeses: cheddar, Edam, Swiss, Stilton, mozzarella	
Cereal products and snacks	
Bread, pasta, rice, oatmeal, flours, sweet biscuit/cookies, cakes, pastries, crackers	Savoury snacks made from potato or corn, such as cheese biscuits, crisps/potato chips, Twiglets, Hula-hoops, etc.
Breakfast cereals: cornflakes, All-bran, and all those made from wheat, rice, oats, and corn	
Miscellaneous	
Margarines, cooking oils	Soya sauce, tomato ketchup, savoury sauces, worcester sauce, gravy mixes, stock cubes
Chocolate and sugar-based confectionery	Yeast extracts (Marmite, Bonox, Vegemite)
Pickled vegetables, vinegar, salad dressings	Meat extracts (Bovril)
Canned puddings, dessert mixes, jellies/gelation desserts, pancake mixes	Fish, meat pastes, pâtés
Sugar, honey, molasses, treacle	Canned and packet soups
Drinks	
Beers, lagers, ciders	Wines, port, liqueurs, sherry
Spirits (whisky, gin, rum)	Tomato juice
Fruit juices, colas, sodas	
Tea, coffee, drinking chocolates, malted drinks (e.g. Ovaltine, Milo, etc.)	

ask the chef or cook whether MSG has been included in the recipe, but the reply you get might be somewhat unreliable! MSG is widely used in Chinese food, and even those restaurants that say they do not use it may use a lot of a particular ingredient with a high level of natural free glutamate, such as soya sauce.

Alternatively, you can opt for a restaurant like the café which serves meals such as fish and chips or steak and potatoes. While this may restrict your choice somewhat, at least you will have the comfort of knowing you won't end the day suffering from Chinese Restaurant Syndrome.

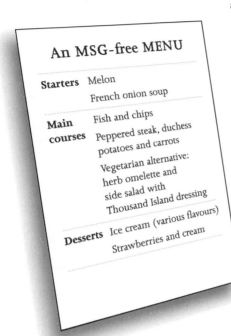

An MSG-free MENU

Starters	Melon
	French onion soup
Main courses	Fish and chips
	Peppered steak, duchess potatoes and carrots
	Vegetarian alternative: herb omelette and side salad with Thousand Island dressing
Desserts	Ice cream (various flavours)
	Strawberries and cream

CHAPTER 2

Alcohol: intoxication and detoxification

On New Year's Day millions of people suffer the symptoms of their body's intolerance of what it regards as too much of a toxin: alcohol. The collection of symptoms they experience—the throbbing headache, the feeling of nausea, even vomiting and diarrhoea—are all typical responses to an excess of a material that the body wishes to be rid of. Our attitude to alcohol is ambivalent: we are prepared to accept the punishment of a hangover because we enjoy the effects that alcohol has on us.

A couple of drinks after a hard day, or with a meal, are very relaxing, and this amount of alcohol does not exceed the limit we can easily detoxify by morning. Intoxication generally occurs at a party when we drink to release ourselves from the inhibitions that normally interfere with social contact. After several drinks, we may find ourselves being friends with everyone around us, laughing and joking and saying outrageous things, and behaving in a manner that we may well wish to forget the next day.

Heavy drinking leads to our most likely experience of intolerance of an alien chemical. Understanding what that chemical is, what it does to us, and how our system deals with it, will help us understand the effects of other common toxicants that come with our food. What is slightly different about alcohol is that our body removes it by turning it first into the chemical that produces all the unpleasant symptoms we experience, and then into a chemical that we can use as a source of energy. This explains the curious nature of alcohol, which acts in three ways:

(1) as a pleasant drink that makes us feel good;

(2) as a toxin, when it is in the first stages of disposal;

(3) as a nutrient, in that it provides our system with energy.

In chemical terms these stages are due to three chemicals: (1) alcohol itself, which is oxidised to acetaldehyde (2), which in turn is oxidised to acetic acid (3). This is finally converted to carbon dioxide and breathed out.

> The alcohol we drink is also known as ethyl alcohol, and its correct chemical name is ethanol.
>
> Acetaldehyde's chemical name is ethanal.
>
> Acetic acid's chemical name is ethanoic acid.

The risks and benefits of drinking alcohol

There are good reasons for *not* consuming alcohol. On health grounds the risks are addiction, illness, and obesity and the problems associated with it. Alcohol provides 700 calories per 100 grams, making it second only to fats and oils which provide 900 calories per 100 g. There are other good reasons in *favour* of consuming alcohol—at least in moderation. It immediately reduces mental stress, and in the long run it benefits the heart. This evidence is based on epidemiological surveys which show the incidence of heart disease is lower among those who follow the guidelines for sensible drinking than among those who do not. These are that a woman should drink no more than three units of alcohol a day, and a man no more than four. We will explore what this means later in this chapter.

Alcohol can be regarded as a form of food. A unit of alcohol (10 g) provides us with about 70 calories of energy. The recommended maximum intake for a man is 28 units of alcohol a week, and this will provide about 2000 calories of his energy needs. For a woman, the recommended amount is 21 units of alcohol, which will provide around 1500 calories. While these are not excessive amounts, they nevertheless must be taken into account when planning a diet. Alcohol accounts for about 10% of the food intake of adults in the USA and Europe. It was once considered such a convenient way of providing energy that it used to be added to intravenous drips as a supplement.

The benefits of alcohol are varied. Some are well known: For example, a nightcap of a glass of beer, or a shot of whisky, can help us get to sleep. However, it may not be a good night's sleep, because alcohol appears to deprive us of a key type of sleep: the early sleep in which we dream. Continued loss of this essential sleep may be the reason why very heavy drinkers eventually suffer hallucinations when it is withheld (traditionally known as the *delirium tremens,* or the 'd.t.s').

Moderate drinkers, those who take two or three units of alcohol a day, gain real advantages. They suffer less coronary heart disease and have lower cholesterol levels. Studies of the life-style of French farmers supports drinking as beneficial, as revealed in the leading medical journal the *Lancet* in 1992. Dr Serge Renaud of the National Institute of Health and Medical Research in Lyons, France, believes that French farmers are less prone to coronary heart disease, despite a diet rich in animal fats, because of their relatively high consumption of alcohol in the form of red wine. Two glasses a day is the recommended amount. Red wine is not a medicine, and it will not cure or relieve heart problems that are already present. If there is any value in drinking red wine, it lies in its ability to prevent heart disease. This message of the benefits of red wine increased sales by over 44% in the USA when it was announced in 1992—perhaps not surprisingly, since almost a million Americans a year die of cardiovascular diseases.

A group at the Kaiser Permanent Medical Center in Oakland, California, claimed that drinkers of white wine were also less likely to suffer coronary heart disease. Whether it is the alcohol itself, or other compounds such as polyphenols in the wine, that are responsible is a matter of debate. A polyphenolic compound called resveratrol has been particularly highlighted as the likely agent, because this is the most abundant: there is up to 3 mg per litre in red wine, but there is very little of it in white wine.

One theory is that the antioxidant behaviour of the polyphenols helps prevent atherosclerosis, keeps blood vessels relaxed, and has an anticoagulant effect. They appear to slow down plaque formation from low-density lipoproteins (LDL), the 'bad' form of cholesterol. When LDL is oxidised it is scavenged by the white blood cells, which remove it from the bloodstream and dump it inside the lining of the arteries. This leads to a build-up of cholesterol in the arteries, which causes narrowing and may ultimately clog them.

Edwin Frankel, a research chemist at the University of California at Davis, reported in 1995 that red wine inhibited LDL oxidation by 46–100%, whereas white wines achieved only 3–6% inhibition. Other work, published in 1996 in the *British Medical Journal,* by Eric Rimm of the Harvard School of Public Health, Boston, USA, suggests that it is the alcohol itself that protects the heart if you have high cholesterol levels, and that this benefit is unrelated to the colour of the wine. Rimm points out that there is overwhelming evidence that alcohol, from whatever source, slows the clotting of blood and increases levels of the high-density lipoproteins (HDL), the 'good' form of cholesterol.

However it works its magic, alcohol certainly seems to reward many of its moderate users; those who drink two units of alcohol a day are reputed to catch half the number of colds that non-drinkers suffer. Nevertheless, there is evidence that drinkers show an increased incidence of cancer of the upper gastrointestinal tract, and in particular of the oesophagus and stomach.

Drink may be beneficial for the heart, only in moderation. Men who drink more than the equivalent of six pints of beer a day (12 units) are twice as likely to suffer a sudden heart attack as non-drinkers, according to Professor Gerry Shaper of the Royal Free Hospital in London, who carried out an eight-year study of over 7500 middle-aged men. Each year about 25 died this way, and two thirds of these were in the heavy-drinking category.

Not everyone is convinced that moderate alcohol consumption is beneficial. At the Novartis Foundation Symposium on Alcohol and Cardiovascular Disease, held in London in October 1997, the epidemiological surveys on which the evidence of beneficial drinking is based were criticised on the basis that they did not properly take into account social status. It was pointed out that moderate drinkers and those who drank wine were more likely to come from the more affluent sections of society, whose health is above average, while heavy drinkers and non-drinkers are usually working-class people, with all the health disadvantages that this status implies.

The composition of alcoholic drinks

Humans have been making, drinking, and recovering from alcohol for almost 7000 years. The earliest evidence for alcohol production was reported by a group of archaeologists from the University of Pennsylvania, who discovered a wine jar in a Neolithic village in the northern Zagros mountains of Iran. Tests showed that it was made in around 5000BC, and it contained traces of tartaric acid, which occurs in large quantities only in grapes, and of oleoresin, which comes from the terebinth tree, and which was used to prevent the growth of microbes that can turn wine into vinegar.

Alcoholic drinks come in a large number of guises, but the main ones are beers, wines, and spirits. What distinguishes the last of these from the other two is the chemical process of distillation, which concentrates and purifies the alcohol. Any sugary solution can be fermented to make alcohol, and in many countries there are drinks produced from a wide variety of plant sugars. Grapes, barley, corn, sugarcane, fruit, potatoes, and rice are all used to make alcoholic drinks. Once these crops have been harvested, and the sugars of the carbohydrates in them have been released, the sugars may be fermented into alcohol by acting as food for yeast. Yeast uses simple sugars in much the same way we do—as a source of energy; but, unlike humans, who generate their energy with the help of oxygen from the air, the yeast generates its energy anaerobically, in other words without oxygen, and the product is alcohol.

Wine can be made simply by crushing grapes, squeezing out the juice, and allowing it to ferment with the wild yeasts that are naturally present on the grapes. This can be a hit-and-miss affair, and does not always produce the desired result. It is better to add the right yeast to the grape juice—the preferred yeast for wine is *Saccharomyces ellipsoideus*. However, this still does not stop millions of litres of wine going to waste because rogue yeasts have outpaced the starter yeast that the vintner added. Some rogue yeasts even produce toxins that can kill the commercial starter yeasts. Not all wild yeasts are bad: some impart a new flavour to the wine, and so are cultured and added to the crushed grape. Wine-makers jealously guard their strains of yeast.

Unwanted bacteria in wine are kept down by using sulfur dioxide, which is added as a solution in water, or as sodium sulfite which dissolves in water and forms sulfur dioxide. In earlier times 'sulfiting' was done simply by burning sulfur near the vat of grape juice. This additive can affect those sensitive to it, as we shall see in Chapter 7, but for some white wines it is an important element of the flavour.

> It always pays to have both red and white wine at dinner. If you spill some of the red wine on the table cloth you can easily remove its stains with the white wine. The sulfur dioxide in the white wine acts as a bleaching agent.

Wine consists of hundreds of chemicals apart from water and alcohol, such as other alcohols, aldehydes, acids, and esters. There are tannins, amino acids, minerals, and aromatic substances. Sparkling wines contain carbon dioxide gas under pressure, and traditionally this is generated in a second fermentation by adding sugar and a pure yeast culture. These bottles are kept clamped tight and left for three to five years while the pressure, builds up. The residual yeast is removed by freezing the neck of the inclined bottle and removing the sediment as an ice plug. This is a time-consuming procedure, and more often now the second fermentation is carried out in steel pressure tanks and the wine is bottled under pressure.

Beer is a different story. The first written accounts of this drink date from the Egypt of the 1st Dynasty, around 3000BC, but there is evidence that ale was first brewed in Babylon about a thousand years earlier. Ale is produced from fermented barley, but the starch in cereal grains can not be fermented by yeasts, which need simple sugars to work on. The first step in brewing ale is to steep the barley in water for a day or two, and then leave it in a warm, damp room for a few more days so that it will germinate. This process is called malting. The grain sprouts develop enzymes that break down the starch into simple sugars. The malted barley is next heated to stop the sprouting and steeped in water to soak out the sugars, which are then fermented.

Adding hops before the fermentation stage imparts flavour and releases preservative chemicals that prevent the growth of bacteria that might spoil the beer. Finally, the yeast *Saccharomyces cerevisiae* is added, and the mixture is left to ferment for a week or so. As the yeast multiplies it produces not only alcohol but also a whole cocktail of organic molecules that give the beer its flavour. Lager is fermented with a different yeast, *Saccharomyces carlsbergensis*.

Distill an alcoholic drink, and it yields a much stronger brew. The art of distillation was discovered by the ancient Romans over 2000 years ago, and brought to a fine art by the monks of the Middle Ages. Distilling wine drives off the alcohol first, and when the vapours, the 'spirits', are cooled and collected you have a product that is mainly ethanol, the alcohol that we drink. In fact small amounts of another alcohol, methanol, may come off first, but this is discarded; then the alcohol we want distils over (it boils at 78 °C). The vapour that condenses also contains some water, but a second and maybe a third distillation will reduce the amount of water to give a product that is 95% alcohol. This is diluted with pure water to around 40% alcohol to make it drinkable. A litre bottle of spirits of normal strength consists of 400 ml of alcohol and 600 ml of distilled water, plus traces of essential extras in tiny amounts.

What distinguishes the different kinds of spirits are these tiny amounts of other volatiles that distil over with the alcohol. Thus we have the distinctive flavours of brandy (which is distilled from wine), whisky (which, like beer, is made from fermented barley), rum (from fermented molasses) and bourbon (from fermented maize). Vodka is made from fermented grain or potatoes, and is the purest drink of all because it is passed through a charcoal filter to remove everything except the alcohol. This is why it is almost tasteless.

In theory, spirits are alcoholic beverages that will do all that beers and wines will do, but which are free of impurities. Spirits act as a preservative, since nothing can live in them; for the same reason, they are also a useful antiseptic when pure. Down the centuries, distilled alcohol has been a part of the medical pharmacopeia. The first distilled alcohol was known as aqua vitae, the water of life, and was valued for its restorative properties. Spirits have also been used by doctors as an anaesthetic, for disinfecting wounds, and for cleaning the skin before injections.

Gin is made from fermented grain alcohol, and is flavoured by a second and even third distillation after herbs, fruits, and berries have been allowed to steep in it. These so-called botanicals must include juniper—this is the essential component that identifies a drink as gin—while the other botanicals may be coriander, angelica, orris root, almonds, cassia bark, liquorice, orange and lemon peel, cardamom, cinnamon, and nutmeg.

The flavour molecules found in Scotch whisky are formed at all stages in its production, and even include some from the peat smoke used to dry the malt. The mashing stage, which extracts the sugars from the malted barley, also extracts other flavours, and the fermentation with yeast produces yet more volatile substances. The final stage in the life of a whisky is its stay in a bonded warehouse for at least three years, although this period may last up to 12 years or more. This ageing leaches out more chemicals from the wood of the cask. All the components are there in minute traces, but are enough to give the drink its characteristic flavour.

Chemical analysis shows there to be some rather surprising natural chemicals in drink, such as dimethyl sulfide, the chemical responsible for bad breath, and hydrogen cyanide (also known as Prussic acid or hydrocyanic acid). This almond-flavoured chemical is there only in a few parts per million—too little to affect us. Another component in much larger amounts is methanol, and this can be worrying. It is possible to end up literally blind drunk on illicit spirits which have high levels of methanol. Our body, turns methanol into formaldehyde and formic acid, a chemical that attacks the retina of the eye. But the low level of methanol in normal wines and spirits is quite harmless.

Alcohol and body chemistry

Although it is naturally always present in our body, alcohol is not there as part of our metabolism, which is the name given to the massive collection of complex chemical reactions that are going on inside all living cells, including those of the human body. A little alcohol is produced from carbohydrates within our intestines by bacteria and yeasts, which have enzymes that can turn carbohydrate into alcohol. This alcohol then passes into our bloodstream. Our liver produces an enzyme called alcohol dehydrogenase (ADH) which we use to get rid of this unwanted chemical, and it turns it first into acetaldehyde. This molecule is also unwanted, so there is another enzyme, acetaldehyde dehydrogenase, which converts it into acetic acid. This is rather a neat way of eliminating the toxin, because it is converted into a chemical the body produces anyway, as part of the mechanism by which it extracts energy from food. This extra source of acetic acid is then put to good use as it is readily oxidised by our tissues to provide energy, and when all its energy has been extracted, it emerges as carbon dioxide from our lungs.

Men can usually tolerate more alcohol than women can. This difference is due to differences in body size and in capacity to absorb the alcohol from the stomach into the bloodstream. Men are generally taller and many pounds heavier than women, and so can spread this chemical over their bigger bodies so that its effect on the brain is less. Also, men have more ADH in their stomach and acetaldehyde production begins there, so that drink-for-drink, less alcohol gets into a man's bloodstream. Native Americans and Oriental people have the same lower level of ADH as women. For such people a couple of drinks is enough to make them tipsy. Once the alcohol is in the bloodstream, men and women are much more alike. The male and female kidneys dispose of alcohol at the same rate, and tests in the USA showed that when men and women were given the same amount of alcohol by injection straight into their bloodstream, there were no sex-related differences in behaviour.

Our liver can deal with quite large amounts of alcohol, if it has to, but it needs time. Meanwhile the alcohol, and the acetaldehyde produced from it, have different effects on parts of the body.

In the brain and central nervous system, alcohol acts as a *depressant*. This does not mean that it makes us depressed. What alcohol does is to slow down brain activity, and slows down messages so they take longer to travel along nerve fibres. We become generally more relaxed and react more slowly, and our speech may even become slurred. Alcohol has this effect because it replaces water molecules around nerve cells, and this interferes with the movement of electric potential along the nerve fibre. Alcohol also slows the movement of the chemical messenger molecules that transmit signals from cell to cell.

Inside the ears are the organs that give us our sense of balance. Alcohol changes the density of the tissue and fluid in them, and the more alcohol we take the bigger the changes become until we lose our normal sense of balance. The result is that when we stand up we feel unsteady, and to compensate for this we sway and stagger around.

Alcohol raises our pulse and blood pressure, but it is the acetaldehyde that produces the warming effect by dilating the blood vessels under our skin, thereby increasing the flow of blood and transfer of body heat to the surface. In the scalp and around the brain this may be part of the reason we end up with a bad headache.

Because men begin to convert alcohol to acetaldehyde, which is an irritant, in their stomach, they should not drink unless they have eaten first—especially if they are prone to ulcers. The presence of fat in the stomach slows down emptying of its contents into the intestines, and this also slows down the absorption of alcohol.

The liver is the main body organ for eliminating alcohol, but it works at a fixed rate which can't be speeded up to deal with a sudden influx of the offending toxin. Indeed, people have been known to fail a breathalyser test 24 hours after their last drink. Alcohol also stimulates the breakdown of glycogen to glucose in the liver, so depleting the body's immediate store of energy.

Alcohol acts as a diuretic: it stimulates the loss of water from the body as urine. If you drink 250 ml of wine (about 2 glasses) you are likely to lose about twice this volume of water as urine during the next two hours. Normally our kidneys will reabsorb and reuse water, and are prompted to do so by a hormone called vasopressin, which is released by the pituitary gland at the base of the brain. Alcohol reduces the amount of vasopressin, and so the kidneys fail to get the message to recycle water, which then passes to the bladder and out of the body. Part of the discomfort of a hangover may be due to dehydration, which is why it is always wise to drink a large glass of water before going to bed if you have been drinking heavily.

All of the above effects are the results of an intolerance reaction to alcohol and acetaldehyde. The result is that we can not avoid feeling ill after taking in too much alcohol, but this is a condition that will cure itself after about 12 hours as our bodily functions return to normal. But alcohol can do serious harm to the human body if we take in too much, too often. We may end up with impaired brain function and memory loss, acute inflammation of the stomach, obesity, addiction, liver disease, a particularly nasty form of heart disease called cardiomyopathy (also known as alcoholic heart muscle disease), and possibly even cancer of the oesophagus. Cardiomyopathy is found in people who have consumed alcohol at the rate of 80 g per day for ten years or more, which is equivalent to drinking a bottle of wine a day. Heavy drinking has been shown to increase the risk of sudden cardiac death, especially among men aged 50 to 60.

The effects of alcohol on the liver are complex and still not clearly understood. They stem from changes in the levels of co-factors, which are chemicals that are necessary to the action of enzymes. The outcome is that the oxidation of fatty acids is impaired in the mitochondria, the parts of cells that generate energy, and so more fats are synthesised. These fats accumulate in the liver to produce what is known as fatty liver, a symptom of alcoholism. Cirrhosis of the liver is a condition in which normal tissue is replaced by collagen (fibrous tissue). As a consequence, the liver functions less efficiently. Cirrhosis is exacerbated by long-term abuse of alcohol. It was once thought to be caused by it, but this now seems unlikely.

Alcoholism is believed to affect about 200 people in 100 000, and is responsible for the deaths of 25 in 100 000 each year in the UK. This condition may be partly inherited, according to studies by Ernest Noble of the University of California, Los Angeles, and Kenneth Blum of the University of Texas. A study on 1033 pairs of identical female twins provided additional proof of a genetic factor. Kenneth Kendler at Virginia Commonwealth University in Richmond reported in the *Journal of the American Medical Association* that the chances of twins both becoming alcoholics were much higher than expected; Kendler suspected that hereditary factors may account for this condition in 60 per cent of cases.

Yet alcohol can be beneficial. In 1997 a 12-year study on 34 000 middle-aged French men, carried out at the University of Bordeaux, concluded that for moderate drinkers there was 30% less cardiovascular diseases. Cancer rates remained the same as for non-drinkers.

Intoxication

If you drink too much alcohol in one session, you may even die. There is a lethal dose of this chemical in an average-sized bottle of spirits. It is difficult to kill yourself this way, but a few people manage it each year. The more usual death from drinking is as a result of driving, and it was this that first led to the discussions about safe limits of intake.

The amount of alcohol in drink can vary widely. A pint of beer (570 ml), which is 5% alcohol by volume, provides around 23 g of alcohol. A glass of wine (125 ml), which is 12% alcohol, contains 12 g, and so does a measure of spirits. These quantities are only rough guides because the amount of alcohol in wine, beer, and spirits can vary markedly. Those who give advice about drinking generally refer to a 'unit' of alcohol, but the definition of this varies from country to country and even within a country. For example, in the UK the British Medical Association defines a unit as 10 g, while the industry and the Government prefer to measure alcohol in volumes, and talk of a unit as 10 ml (which is around 8 g). In the USA the unit is 12 g and in Canada it is 13 g.

Table 2.1 The effects of alcohol.

Units	No. of drinks			Blood level (mg/100 ml)	Effects on average man[a]
	beer	wine	spirits		
2	1 pint	2 glasses	2 singles	30	feels good
4	2 pints	half bottle	2 doubles	50	uninhibited
8	4 pints	bottle	4 doubles	100	unsteady
16	8 pints	2 bottles	1/2 bottle	250	drunk
24	12 pints	3 bottles	3/4 bottle	400	dead drunk

[a]For a woman, the same effects may be experienced with about two thirds the amount of alcohol that a man needs.

The effects of drinking alcohol can be seen in Table 2.1. This table can not take into account all the factors that determine the effect that alcohol will have, because this depends on a person's weight, the condition of their liver, and whether the alcohol is taken with a meal.

Detoxification

Alcohol passes from the gut into the bloodstream and is then circulated around the body. Ten per cent of it escapes without being absorbed because it is exhaled on our breath, sweated through our pores, or passed out in our urine. The other 90% is eventually processed by the liver, which can deal with 12 ml (10 g) of alcohol an hour. While the effect of this is to lower the body's level of alcohol, and so sober us up, it thereby increases the body's burden of acetaldehyde, which takes just as long to remove. This explains the effects we experience when we drink heavily at a party. To begin with, we take in alcohol at a rate much faster than the ADH enzyme can remove it, and we enjoy the pleasures of intoxication. Meanwhile, the level of acetaldehyde is increasing, but we don't notice this since it is masked by the effects of the alcohol. Eventually we stop drinking, and generally we go to sleep. Slowly the level of alcohol falls, while that of acetaldehyde continues to climb, until we awake in the morning when this toxin now dominates, and we have a hangover. But help is already at hand: a second enzyme, acetaldehyde dehydrogenase, is already working to remove the acetaldehyde and slowly it succeeds. By the afternoon most of this toxin will have disappeared, and we will feel better.

The term 'detoxification' is commonly misused to suggest that we, as individuals, have some control over our body's metabolism for removing unpleasant substances that serve no useful purpose, and may actually harm us. So-called 'detox' dietary regimes are based on the erroneous idea that the body is clogged up with all kinds of harmful and unnatural 'chemicals' that need to be flushed out of the system. Colonic irrigation does this literally—but to no real effect. Other detox treatments focus on the other end of the gut and are based on dietary regimes. These will have a real benefit if they persuade us to correct bad eating habits, restrain from excessive drinking of alcohol, cut down on caffeine, or stop smoking. The simple expedient of drinking only water, eating only fruit at every meal for a few days, and going for long walks, would improve the health of most people who are overweight and under-exercised. Such a regime can be seen as detoxification, but it is not detoxification in the way the body knows it.

The body's detoxification mechanism is working all the time, and it relies on *enzymes* to destroy those chemicals in our food that threaten us. Enzymes are protein structures capable of changing a chemical from one form to another, and they are usually specific in the changes they can make. Enzymes are there to digest our food, extract energy from it, build up new molecules for the cells of our body, carry out essential functions, and keep our nerves and senses working. Enzymes are even needed to make other enzymes.

The enzymes used for detoxification lie in wait, but if there is a sudden excess of toxic molecules to be dealt with then the body needs to be able to manufacture enough enzymes to meet the threat. It is relatively easy to overwhelm the body's detoxification mechanisms with alcohol and acetaldehyde, because the enzymes that deal with these work by a 'zero-order' process. If they operated by a 'first-order' process there would be much less of a problem.

When enzyme activity increases in line with the extent of the threat, we call this a 'first-order' process, which is a technical term based on chemical reactivity. Not all enzymes respond this way. Some can only work at a fixed rate, which is independent of the amount of toxin there is to be dealt with, and this is called a 'zero-order' process. Sadly for us, most detoxification works like this. Our bodies have evolved to meet a certain level of natural toxicants and non-nutrients that are present in our food, and we feel no adverse effects from eating them. When we suddenly take in too much, then the body simply has to live with the excess until the offending substance can be removed. It is the *excess* that explains the symptoms of intolerance.

Sometimes we can prolong the agony of alcohol detoxification by blocking the enzyme acetaldehyde dehydrogenase with a drug, which does not appear to be a wise thing to do, but it can be done as a way of discouraging those who have become addicted to alcohol and persuading them to stay off drink. Antabuse is that type of drug, as the box explains.

The Antabuse story

Antabuse was discovered in Denmark during World War II, when Dr Jens Hald was researching a treatment for intestinal worms. A chemical called disulfiram had been used successfully to treat the parasitic skin disease scabies, and when Hald tested disulfiram on rabbits infected with worms, it appeared to cure them. To test whether it was safe for humans to take, he then began to take the drug himself, and so did his colleague Dr Erik Jacobsen. They each took a disulfiram pill every day for several weeks. Most days they were fine, but on some days they suffered a severe reaction, headache, vomiting, and flushing, which generally happened in the afternoon.

Then one evening Hald shared a bottle of cognac with a friend. He quickly became very ill, while his friend was fine. Hald then realised that previous attacks coincided with lunches at which he had drunk alcohol. When he told Jacobsen, he too confirmed that his intolerance reactions were linked to his drinking alcohol. Tests on volunteers confirmed that this was so, and disulfiram was dropped as a possible treatment for worms.

That might have been the end of the matter, but after the war, in 1947, Jacobsen told the disulfiram story as an amusing aside at a meeting he was addressing. A journalist from the Copenhagen newspaper *Berlingske Tidende* was present, and reported the story. Alcoholics who read about disulfiram realised that here was a treatment that might wean them off alcohol, and several of them wrote to Jacobsen, asking for disulfiram tablets. Clinical tests on alcoholic volunteers showed that the drug could be used to break the addiction to alcohol. Antabuse, the trade name Jacobsen gave the drug, was launched.

People who are addicted to alcohol and really want to break their addiction can take a regular dose of Antabuse, and they then think twice before succumbing to the temptation to drink alcohol because the effects are so unpleasant.

Antabuse works by blocking the enzyme that converts acetaldehyde to acetic acid. A build-up of acetaldehyde produces a condition known as acetaldehydemia, which can be violently unpleasant. Even a little alcohol taken by someone on Antabuse produces enough acetaldehyde for their body to react unpleasantly to it. They feel very ill because they are in effect experiencing a severe hangover, the symptoms of which are nausea, vomiting, laboured breathing, flushing, chest pains, and throbbing headache. The experience is so dreadful that they will usually avoid alcohol while they remain on Antabuse, although it has been found that some people can become tolerant of the drug and its effect is diminished. Most people who take Antabuse find it effective; but they must also be alert to the fact that some common household products contain alcohol, such as vanilla extract (35% alcohol), cough medicines (up to 25% alcohol), and mouthwashes (around 25% alcohol).

Alcohol can interfere with the body's ability to detoxify other chemicals it wishes to be rid of. Alcohol detoxification ties up the enzymes of one of the metabolic pathways used for breaking down the amine serotonin. Because serotonin is a powerful transmitter in the brain, it may be the increased levels of it that are responsible for the feel-good effects that occur when we have something to drink. We shall look at this in more detail in Chapter 4.

The morning after and how to avoid it

Once alcohol is absorbed by our body we have to contend first with its effects, and later with those of its by-product acetaldehyde. This acetaldehyde is the most likely cause of our hangover: it is known to cause headaches and nausea. Dehydration may add to our misery. Is it possible to neutralise the effects of alcohol? In other words, can we take something that will immediately sober us up? Will it also neutralise the effects of the acetaldehyde that will be produced as the alcohol is detoxified?

Since there is no known way of boosting the amount of the detoxifying enzyme, ADH, that our body produces, there can be no 'instant' cure to sober us up. The popular remedies of sweating in a sauna, vigorous exercise, drinking black coffee, and putting your head under the cold tap are all ineffective. Nor is there a successful hangover cure, because again there is no known way of boosting levels of the acetaldehyde dehydrogenase that will speed up the removal of the excess acetaldehyde from the body. The traditional remedy for a hangover is : 'the hair of the dog that bit you'—in other words, have another drink. This will only be of relief if you are addicted to alcohol, in which case the unpleasant effects of your hangover are mainly withdrawal symptoms. One popular hangover preventative consists of the painkiller paracetamol, citric acid, sodium and potassium bicarbonates, and vitamin C. A sachet of this in water is to be taken before going to bed, and the dose repeated on waking. Clearly this will go some way to alleviating the hangover symptoms of a headache and an upset stomach.

But all we can really do is try to delay the absorption of alcohol when we start drinking, and to alleviate the symptoms of acetaldehyde when we are recovering from a hangover. The following suggestions may relieve the worst excesses of both these chemicals:

- Have a glass of milk before you start drinking, so that you are not drinking on an empty stomach.
- Stick to one type of alcoholic drink, and occasionally have a soft drink.
- Drink a pint of water before going to bed to counter dehydration.
- For breakfast eat something sweet, such as honey or jam. These foods contain a lot of fructose, which is the sugar that generates nicotinamide adenine dinucleotide (NAD), a co-factor involved in the detoxification of alcohol. Extra sugar will also help restore the body's depleted glycogen store.
- Avoid drinks such as sherry, which contain histamine. As we shall see in Chapter 4, this is also a hidden danger in our diet.

Enzymes and detoxification

In this chapter we have seen how two enzymes, alcohol dehydrogenase and acetaldehyde dehydrogenase, are waiting to detoxify any alcohol that come their way. In this respect our defences against alcohol are rather specialised. Generally it is not worthwhile for the body to produce a specific enzyme for each likely toxin. Instead, it relies on a few enzymes that can aid the excretion of unwanted molecules by making them more soluble, so that they can more easily be removed via the kidneys and urine.

Essential to most detoxification is a system called the cytochrome-P450 pathway, which was first uncovered in the late 1950s as the way amphetamines were detoxified. Since then a lot of scientific work has been conducted on this incredibly versatile system. The enzyme cytochrome-P450 is present in all animal species, and in mammals it has two functions: making hormones and detoxifying unwanted chemicals. This latter role is thought to have its origin in the survival of animal species that evolved P450 as a defence against plant toxins. Its prime quality is its ability to engage a large number of different substances (termed 'substrates'), and this is why it can detoxify a wide range of poisons. But this versatility comes at a price: it has a slower turnover and is less efficient than other systems. Moreover, different people produce different amounts of P450, which is why some people have little difficulty detoxifying some chemicals, while others can be overwhelmed by them.

Detoxification mechanisms work by making potentially toxic substances less soluble in fat. The chemistry is like that of a French salad dressing made from olive oil, wine vinegar, lemon juice, salt, pepper, garlic and sugar. These are shaken thoroughly in a bottle to form an emulsion that mixes all the flavours, but if it is left to stand for a while the contents will settle out into two layers with the watery ingredients at the bottom (vinegar and lemon juice) and the olive oil at top. The sugar and salt will be dissolved in the water layer, whereas the flavour molecules from the garlic and pepper will dissolve in the oil.

The same separation into water-soluble and fat-soluble components happens in the human body. Fat-soluble molecules will dissolve in the fatty tissues of the body. If these molecules are toxins, we need to eliminate them via the blood, so they have to be converted to water-soluble molecules. Once they are dissolved in the blood, the toxin molecules can be excreted in the urine or dumped in the lower gut to form part of the faeces. The P450 system converts fat-soluble into water-soluble molecules by inserting an oxygen atom into each toxic molecule, producing an hydroxyl group which has a greater affinity for water than for fat.

The first step in this detoxification process requires the unwanted molecule to be caught by the P450 system's enzymes. This is done at a receptor site that can trap and hold the molecule while it is oxidised, a process that takes about ten seconds. Nine steps are involved in this process, during which electrons are lost and replaced, and oxygen is brought in, activated, and then added to the molecule to form the hydroxyl group. The molecule is then expelled by the enzyme, which can then repeat the process when it encounters another toxin molecule. Ten seconds may sound quite quick for the complex job the P450 is doing, but it is slow compared to the speed with which many other enzyme systems operate. If the body has to deal with billions and trillions of toxic molecules, then speed becomes critical if disposal is to succeed at a faster rate than the toxin can wreak its damage.

It does not matter to the P450 system whether the compounds to be oxidised are simple molecules, or complex ones, or whether they contain sulfur, nitrogen, halogens, or other complex chemical groups. It can deal with them all. While the system is versatile, it does have a fixed rate of action, and so overload is always a possibility. To cope with this there are enzyme back-up systems to hold the offending toxins until the load is lessened and they can be dealt with. These holding enzymes bind the toxin to proteins or to scavenging white cells in the blood, which can transport the toxins to the organs where detoxification occurs. In some instances, these back-up systems can actually start the detoxification process themselves.

Some people are much better at detoxifying unwanted molecules than are other members of their family, friends, and neighbours, which is why they can react very differently to the same meal. Some people can detoxify unwanted components four times faster than other people. Moreover, illness can reduce an individual's ability to detoxify to a third of normal, and this happens with even mild illnesses like the common cold. Thus there can be a twelve-fold difference in the rate at which a healthy fast-metabolising individual can detoxify a poison compared to a slow metaboliser who is not well. Now we can understand why there is so much variation in the way people react to various chemicals.

Considering the wide range of chemicals used today as drugs and food additives, and the efficient way the body utilises and eliminates them, you might wonder how we evolved to anticipate having to cope with all these new chemical entities that modern humans encounter. The answer of course is that defence mechanisms have long been in place for dealing with the natural non-nutrients and toxins, the so-called xenobiotics, that are present in food. The P450 system and associated enzymes are so versatile that almost any unwanted molecule, natural or manufactured, can be targeted and eliminated; nevertheless there are a few exceptions: some compounds are so poisonous that they can not be countered no matter how efficient our detoxification system is. These we have to be taught to avoid. Happily for us, there are relatively few of them.

CHAPTER 3

The gut, the bad, and the allergy

We need all kinds of nutrients to build and repair our body structures. Food also has to provide the necessary energy to bring these processes about, which is why most of our food consists of high energy molecules such as sugars, starch, fats, and oils. Energy is our primary need, but without protein, vitamins, minerals, and a few other molecules we would not be able to extract this energy, which is why a balanced diet is so important.

The tube which runs from the mouth to the anus is called the gastro intestinal tract. The minute food enters our mouths the digestive process begins, deconstructing food into its various components. The selection of what is needed, the rejection of what is not, and the elimination of the waste products of metabolism continue down its length. In the lower, or large bowel, bacteria extract the final amounts of energy and it is these microbes that make up a large part of the stool.

Our gut has a battery of enzymes waiting to digest the carbohydrate, fats, and proteins we consume. These enzymes split the complex food molecules into simpler units that our body can absorb. For example, if we eat a hamburger we make use of its plentiful supply of meat protein, which is the muscle fibre from cattle. Our body may take this protein to make our own muscles; but first it has to be broken down into its component molecules, the amino acids. This is carried out by protease enzymes. When these have done their job, the amino acids penetrate the gut wall and are carried to where they can be used to build not only our muscles but also lots of other body parts as well. They assemble themselves into our body protein according to a formula that is encoded in our genes.

When we digest our food, our body also has to cope with the non-nutrients that accompany the nutrients. The majority of non-nutrients are natural—synthetic chemical additives account for only a small proportion of them—and, by and large, they are non-toxic and beneficial, preserving or enhancing the quality of food and drink.

Any chemical which enters our body—be it a nutrient, trace element or non-nutrient—may be essential, beneficial, inert, or have some pharmacological activity. (Non-nutrients are also known as xenobiotics.) This activity may be quite mild at low doses, but produce a toxic reaction at high doses. For example, vitamin A is an essential component of our diet, but too much provokes a toxic response, and in excess it can be life-threatening. Some xenobiotics produce only a toxic response, no matter what the dose, and the more we take, the more we suffer.

It is important to judge the toleration level for a pharmaceutical compound, since these compounds are designed to have a profound effect on some parts of the body. Those who produce such drugs need to know the ideal therapeutic dose, and research is undertaken in which ever-increasing amounts are given to animals, up to and including lethal doses. From these results it is possible to calculate what will be the safe dose for humans. Even when this has been worked out, a doctor still has to take his patient's individual circumstances into consideration when prescribing the drug.

Food components, whether they be nutrients or non-nutrients, can also provoke a toxic response in our body.

There is an ancient saying that 'one man's meat is another man's poison,' and there is some truth in this observation. There are several reasons why our body may react to food as if it were a poison. It might be because:

(1) a component in it has overwhelmed the body's detoxification mechanisms;

(2) we have over-stimulated our body's receptors with naturally occurring amines;

(3) essential food components have been degraded into toxins by micro organisms; or

(4) our gut wall has been damaged, and lets toxic materials pass through.

All these effects may make us ill. Understanding how and why this happens may help us realise why some foods affect us the way they do.

Coping with toxins

The two most common responses to too much toxin are vomiting and diarrhoea. Vomiting is one of the most primitive functions in most animals, but it does not necessarily indicate poisoning as there are many circumstances that cause it. Over-eating, unpleasant sights, and imminent death may provoke vomiting. Even so, the most likely cause is that the body wishes to rid itself of an excess of a toxin.

Despite being so common, and despite its clinical importance, the act of vomiting is not well understood. In their book *Serotonin and the Scientific Basis of Anti-emetic Therapy,* John Reynolds, Paul Andrews, and Christopher Davis, speak of a possible centre in the brain that triggers vomiting. They claim that this centre, known as the *area postrema,* can be controlled by the neurotransmitter serotonin, and blocked in its action by drugs that are antagonists to serotonin. Since vomiting is an unpleasant side-effect of the chemotherapy used in the treatment of cancer, serotonin antagonist drugs have provided great relief for chemotherapy patients.

The other mechanism for rapidly expelling unwanted material from the gut is diarrhoea. Stools become fluid and frequent, but a side-effect of this is that the body may become dehydrated—a problem that is especially threatening to the lives of babies and young children. Diarrhoea usually is a belated response to milder types of toxins, and happens after the offending material has passed through the stomach. The lower, large bowel accepts very fluid, semi-digested material from the small bowel, and then proceeds to extract from it water, carbohydrates, and other material that has been produced by bacteria. The contractions of the large bowel (peristalsis) move the increasingly solid stool along, and delivers it to the rectum. When the rectum is full, it signals the need to evacuate. Diarrhoea accelerates the whole process, but once the body has rid itself of the unwanted material it will generally settle down to a regular routine again. If a person experiences chronic diarrhoea, then they are likely to lose weight and to become deficient in certain nutrients, and may then need replacement therapy and supplements. They will need to eat more fibre and fat, drink more water, abstain from caffeine, and stop smoking. Drugs may also be given to slow down bowel motion.

Vomiting and diarrhoea are the normal responses of a healthy gut to too much of a toxin. However, in some cases the gut can not perform as efficiently, and the toxins may make us ill. For example wheat, cow's milk, and beans are three common staple foods in our diet, and are eaten by millions with no ill effects. But for some people, these foods are extremely dangerous, and a cause of ill-health. At the time of weaning, babies start on the road to a normal healthy adult diet, and are introduced to new foods usually in sequence. One of the first is cow's milk. At this stage, about one in 2500 babies will start to have a change in bowel habit, often with diarrhoea, colic, eczema, and chronic running nose. They fail to thrive, and start losing weight. Parents become stressed as the baby becomes more and more irritable, and as the symptoms—including abdominal distention and further failure to gain weight—become worse.

Examination of the small bowel in these babies reveals quite marked changes, and the cause seems to be that a damaged gut wall has enabled one of the protein constituents in milk, β-lactoglobulin, to be absorbed in excessive quantities—enough to trigger the body's-defence mechanisms. It is still not clear whether this is due to a bout of gastroenteritis or to a genetic factor; but the result is that the body creates local antibodies in the gut wall, and these combine with the β-lactoglobulin to cause more damage. A vicious circle of further damage, leading to more absorption of the offending material, is set in motion. Removal of cow's milk from the baby's diet usually leads to complete recovery.

Another chemical in milk can also upset the gut and produce almost identical results, but this time by an entirely different mechanism. The offending molecule is the carbohydrate, lactose. Intolerance of lactose may be due to a genetic disorder which means that the body fails to produce an enzyme to digest it, or it may be due to gastroenteritis. When damage occurs to the gut wall, this depresses the levels of all the enzymes that break down carbohydrate into simpler sugars, but lactase, the enzyme for digesting lactose, is depressed more than most. The resulting build-up of undigested material prevents water being absorbed from the gut, and encourages microbes to flourish. These microbes can produce lactic and acetic acids, which irritate the gut wall.

An almost identical pattern of illness can be seen in babies who become sensitive to the gluten protein in wheat and rye. In certain areas, such as the west of Ireland, there is a high incidence of 1 in 300 children who are affected. Unlike the milk sensitivity, this condition can also develop in later life, and there are cases in which patients are not diagnosed until they are over 60. The illness is called coeliac disease, and it means the individual must avoid gluten for life. Nowadays gluten-free products are widely available, though they are somewhat expensive.

Coeliac disease

The physician Galen described the symptoms of coeliac disease at the time of the Roman Empire, but could do little to treat it. In the nineteenth century it was known as nontropical sprue, and still no progress had been made towards a cure. And so things remained until the middle of the twentieth century.

In the 1940s a Dutch pediatrician, Willem-Karo Dicke (1905–1962), began trials with children who were suffering the condition. He put them on wheat-free diets, a regime that was relatively easy in the years when food was rationed. In 1950 his thesis, entitled 'Coeliac disease and the effect of certain cereals' was published by the University of Utrecht, and became world renowned. Further research followed, and today the cause has been narrowed to the gliadin fraction of gluten. People with coeliaec disease, which is more correctly called gluten-sensitive enteropathy, are given professional advice on what to avoid, but rice, corn, fruit, fresh meat, cheese, fats, and oils are fine. They must always be aware that processed foods may contain ingredients derived from grains containing gluten.

The gut wall barrier

The gut is a huge organ, and there are two major problems it has to cope with. First, the small intestine must obtain 50% of the energy it needs to function from the food actually present in it. For the large intestine, this rises to 80% or more. Although it is deep inside us, the gut wall provides a complicated barrier between the body and the outside world. Until something crosses the gut barrier into the tissues and bloodstream, it is regarded as external to the body. The function of the gut is to break down food into the simple molecules that it can absorb, but it must also keep out unwanted substances, towards which it acts as an almost impenetrable barrier. Thus the gut's second major problem is that it must let the nutritional parts of food through the gut wall, while at the same time neutralising or limiting the amount of natural toxins, the xenobiotics, that penetrate it; and it must exclude completely any microbes.

The gut performs these functions very efficiently when we are fit and well, but after an operation or a trauma, or when we are ill or starving, the gut wall can quickly start to atrophy. If we eat nothing at all, this atrophying becomes noticeable after one week. Even in a time of minor illness the gut will malfunction, resulting in a loss of appetite, feeling of nausea, discomfort, and a change in bowel habit.

The gut wall is coated with a sticky mucous, which is released by special cells called goblet cells. These contain local antibodies IgA and IgM, which protect against viruses, bacteria, and toxins. In addition there are enzymes and active chemicals with similar functions. The goblet cells are some of the first to be damaged by disease, diminishing this important part of the gut barrier system.

Simple food molecules are easily absorbed high up in the gut. The more complex molecules require a series of enzymes to break them down to useable units, and the most complex of all require the assistance of the host bacteria that live in the large bowel. These bacteria take complex fibres and proteins, and produce short chain fatty acids and certain amino acids that are capable of providing energy locally to the gut. Gut bacteria are so important to us that they supply us with 25% of our energy needs by digesting carbohydrates and long-chain sugars. This is one reason why the inappropriate use of antibiotics should be discouraged: they kill off these bacteria as well as the bacteria that cause disease.

Although bacteria are extremely beneficial in the gut, if the gut wall is damaged and they cross into the body, then serious illness follows. Bengmark and his colleagues have suggested special diets for those who have suffered gut damage and these are high in oats, which are rich in membrane lipids, and water soluble fibre that is also fermentable, plus beneficial amino acids. These foods do not encourage the growth of gut bacteria, and so reduce the chances of them invading the body and making us ill.

The extent to which the gut wall will allow material to pass through into the bloodstream can be measured using sugar molecules of varying sizes which are not digested. In this way medical scientists have been able to demonstrate how the permeability of the gut varies in a number of conditions. If the gut becomes more permeable, then larger molecules that are normally excluded may get through, and some of these may be toxic, or induce a host reaction in the form of an immune response. The effect may be localised, but in certain instances it may result in a general toxic or allergic response. Irrespective of where the immune response occurs, the body then starts treating the invading molecules as foreign and hostile, and attempts to destroy them. Thus a perfectly harmless food component may become a target for elimination. The result may be a local inflammatory response which damages the gut further, thereby making it even more permeable.

Lymphocyte cells, which are the cornerstone of the body's defence system, build up in massive quantities just under the surface in the gut wall, giving rise to clumps that are called Peyers patches. Lymphocytes become activated to attack a foreign, potentially hostile, invader by learning to recognise part of its molecular structure, and they are able to remember this information and store it in case of future invasions. They can also pass this information on to other lymphocytes, and in this way the body builds a defence system against invading microbes and toxic materials. These activated groups of lymphocytes can now specifically manufacture antibodies which will act as a local defence force. Tiny particles of food that pass through the gut wall before they have been fully digested may also be attacked by lymphocytes and remembered, and attacked again in the future, should they breach the gut wall barrier. Hans Strobel, at the Great Ormond Street Hospital for Sick Children in London, has developed this theory further. According to Strobel, cells with lymphocytes are programmed either to tolerate or to react—and he believes that this is literally vital. The gut wall barrier is the critical factor, not only for deciding which foods will not be tolerated, but also, during development in childhood, enabling the body to decide which foreign material to absorb and use for nutrition.

P. D'Eufemia, of the Institute of Pediatrics of the University of Rome, has studied autistic children, and has noted that their gut is more permeable to larger molecules. Peptides, which are chains of amino acids like proteins, but much shorter, might be a factor in this condition. Increased permeability to molecules such as these also leads to disruption of transport mechanisms across the barrier and to depletion of minerals, vitamins and trace elements, all of which exacerbate the condition.

Eating for a healthy gut

To keep the gut working properly we need to eat a varied diet that provides us with a balance of nutrients. The Appendix explains what these nutrients are and how much of them we need. Alternatively if we have an inadequate diet, or are prone to food fads, or we take in an excess of toxic materials of the kind described in this book, then perhaps we should not be surprised if our gut struggles to perform its normal functions.

Those with irritable bowel syndrome exhibit a common collection of symptoms: wind, bloating, abdominal pain, and changes in bowel habit, such as a change from constipation to loose motions, and vice versa. These symptoms can occur intermittently and mildly, or be of such severity as to dominate a person's daily life. When the symptoms have been fully investigated, and all major bowel ailments have been ruled out, then the condition is referred to as 'irritable bowel syndrome'—but this diagnosis is almost an admission that medical science doesn't know what to do to help. Often a doctor will tell the patient to 'go away and live with it'. Or the advice might be to avoid hot and spicy foods, and while this may do some good, it would be much better to investigate other components of the patient's diet. Then it may be discovered that the patient will respond to changes.

Table 3.1 lists the things that irritate the gut, ranging from the unavoidable to the easily avoided. The list does not include poor nutrition, but if this is also part of a person's way of eating, then there is a recipe for chronic illness. The worst possible approach to irritable bowel syndrome is to embark on a series of novel diets, bizarre supplements, unproven treatments, and ineffectual techniques. These may simply make matters worse. There is no

Table 3.1 The things that can irritate our gut.

Drugs	antibiotics, anti-inflammatory drugs, laxatives, corticosteroids, contraceptive and other hormones, digoxin
Irritants	alcohol and caffeine
Organisms	*Dientamoeba fragilis*, *Blastocystis hominis*, *Giardia lambli*, *Cryptosporidium*, *Helicobacter pylori*, *Klebsiell*, *Citrobacter*
Food additives	dyes, preservatives, peroxidised fats
Enzyme deficiencies	coeliac disease, lactase deficiency
Refined carbohydrate	sweets and chocolates, confectionery, soft drinks, white bread
Natural toxins	moulds, fungi, bacteria, and toxins in fish and honey

point consuming lots of unnecessary, and expensive, dietary aids, if a few more appropriate ones would be more beneficial.

Perhaps one of the more unexpected items that causes bowel disorders is refined carbohydrate, such as sugar. If there is a large excess of sugar at the point in the bowel where it is broken down, it can ferment, producing not only ethanol, the normal alcohol of alcoholic drinks, but also other alcohols such as propanol and butanol, which are more toxic.

The mechanisms that lead to food intolerance are common to all of us, but our response may be very individual. It is food intolerance that accounts for many of the disorders of our gut, even when we are eating food we are familiar with. Sometimes, and without being aware of it, we may overload our body with a particular common toxin, and suffer the consequences. In analysing our body's response to this toxin we may come to focus on one ingredient of what we have just eaten, and believe thereafter that this is something we are *allergic* to and should henceforth avoid. But we may simply have suffered a form of mild poisoning by some natural toxin or non-nutrient in our food.

Food intolerance and food allergy

Food consists of nutrients and non-nutrients. We can be allergic to nutrients, and intolerant of non-nutrients. The way we respond to these threats lies in our genes.

The genetic difference between humans and chimpanzees may be less than 2% of our genetic makeup, but that 2% makes us a distinctly different primate. We have been able to adapt to almost any environment, be it the frozen wastes of the Arctic, the scorching deserts of Arabia, or the high altitudes of Nepal. In all these places humans have bred, survived and flourished, despite the extremes of climate. Part of that adaptation is the ability to use the local food sources of these very different environments as complete nutrition. For example, the women of the Gambia have very little in the way of dairy products, compared to their Finnish counterparts, who enjoy a high dairy intake rich in the calcium that is needed to build strong bones. Yet Gambian women have equally strong bones, because they are able to utilise the small supply of calcium in their diet very efficiently.

Human survival in these very different regions depended on our adapting to a wide variety of foods. To be allergic to a particular food would be a biological disaster, and any who were thus afflicted would have died before they had time to grow up and reproduce, ensuring that this defect in their genetic makeup was not passed on to the next generation. This is why an aberrant or idiosyncratic response to food that we call allergy is so uncommon.

All allergy is genetically predisposed, and is caused by exposure to an allergen, usually one that is very common in a particular environment. In the case of pollen, the Scandinavians become sensitized to silver birch, the British to grass, and the North Americans to ragweed, because those are the plants that prevail in those areas. The more common the allergen, the more likely it will be that some people in the general population will respond badly to it because of their genetic make-up.

So it is with food: the more common the allergen, the more susceptible people are likely to be. Thus cow's milk is more likely to be implicated in allergy, along with other common

foods like wheat, rather than less common foods. A good example of this is peanut sensitivity. This was unheard of in the UK 50 years ago, but as this food has become more popular,
to the extent that it is now imported on a large scale and used in all kinds of products, so the
incidence of acute allergic reactions has risen. People who are allergic can be at risk in many
ways. A recent death from peanut allergy was caused not by eating the nuts, which the
patient assiduously avoided, but from eating chips with a curry sauce that had been made
using cheap groundnut oil. But despite the fact that the number of cases of peanut allergy is
increasing, it is still very rare.

About 90% of food allergies are caused by proteins in certain foods, particularly milk,
eggs, fish, crab, shrimp, lobster, peanuts, tree nuts, soybeans, and wheat. In the USA between
100–200 people die each year from food allergy, which is fewer than one in 10 000 of those
who are allergic. The vast majority of people (99%) are not allergic to their food, although
many may be intolerant of something in their diet. Children are more prone to food allergy,
but most grow out of this as their gut develops and becomes less permeable to the proteins
that trigger the allergic response. In some cases, specific food proteins have been identified
as causing food allergy, such as lactoglobulins in milk, ovomucoid and apovitellins in eggs,
and tropomyosin in shrimp.

An allergic response is not related to the *amount* of the allergen that we consume—a tiny
quantity can trigger a severe reaction. But there is a direct link between the amount of non-
nutrient eaten and the way our body responds to it, especially if the non-nutrient is toxic.
The more of the non-nutrient we take in, the more our body has to dispose of, and if we take
in too much then we can swamp our defences and become ill. As with all toxins, there are
degrees of danger and degrees of the body's ability to deal with the poison. But attempts to
avoid non-nutrients that provoke a toxic response are misguided, unless we know we are
particularly sensitive to them. Indeed, it might even be beneficial to take in small amounts
of such non-nutrients to keep our detoxification defences on the alert.

One chemical that can provoke food intolerance also has a key role in allergic response,
and that is histamine. This is a naturally occurring amine that is produced in the body, but
which needs to be carefully controlled. There are mechanisms for doing this, but we can
have too much histamine, either because we have eaten a food that contains lots of it—and
we shall be dealing with this in Chapter 4, when we consider histamine intolerance—or
because we have a massive release of histamine from our body's own cells. This can happen
as a response to something we are allergic to. When this allergen is eaten, the body releases
massive amounts of histamine into the bloodstream, which is out of all proportion to the
amount of allergen ingested. We then suffer a violent reaction to this essential but unpleasant molecule, which is also toxic in excess.

Testing for allergy

An individual who is allergic to a food will have a demonstrable reaction in that they will
produce the allergic antibody known as immunoglobulin when they eat it. The foods that
cause allergy are quite common, they are usually nutrients, and the agents responsible are
large molecules that are uniquely identifiable. The reaction to them is often very quick, and

may be local or generalised. The local reaction might include swelling where the food is in contact with lips, tongue, mouth, and throat, a condition known as angioneurotic oedema. General reactions such as vomiting, precipitous diarrhoea, streaming nose, and wheezing may follow, and, in extreme cases, circulation and respiration may fail, and the person dies. A patient will be aware of their allergy, knowing that this defence mechanism is a threat to their well-being, and that ingestion, contact, or even odour can trigger an acute response.

The immunological changes associated with allergy are complex, and many of the mechanisms are still not fully researched or understood. The simplest mechanism, however, is well understood, and is called Type 1 immediate hypersensitivity. Antibodies can be measured, and the body produces a variety of them, classified as A, E, G, and M. The immunoglobulin E (IgE) is a rogue antibody, only present in any quantity in patients who suffer from allergic diseases. (The other immunoglobulin antibodies, IgG, IgM, and IgA are all protective and present in all of us.) Each IgE is quite specific to a particular allergen although some allergens produce the same IgE, e.g. fruit, nuts and latex. It combines with the food (the allergen) and the two react with sensitised cells, bursting them open and releasing free histamine, as well as many other compounds that produce the acute effects. This antibody/antigen reaction can be demonstrated in the laboratory using an allergic patient's blood containing the allergic antibodies.

Histamine is used in clinics throughout the world to test for allergy. A drop is placed on the skin and the skin is scratched with a needle through the drop. Within seconds the skin begins to weal and flare, and this acts as a standard against which to compare that person's reaction to other possible allergens such as pollens, dusts, animal danders, and moulds. In the same test, these substances will cause similar weals and flaring if the person is allergic to them.

A negative control and a positive control enable a comparison to be made of an individual's reactions to a series of allergens. The procedure for testing requires the skin to be pricked twice, once with a solution that contains the allergen (the positive), and once with a solution with no allergen (the negative). Sometimes wealing happens with the negative too, but only if a person has very sensitive skin. Sometimes the positive fails to register, and this may happen if the patient has taken an anti-histamine drug before the skin tests.

An allergy clinic will hold several hundred allergens in stock: some from the workplace, some naturally found in the home, some from the environment, and some common foods known to cause reactions via this mechanism. The commonest allergies tend to be to the most prevalent protein complexes to which the allergic individual is exposed, and this is why cows' milk, which is the first food a weaned baby comes across, has caused so much allergy in the form of eczema, bowel disorders, asthma, and running nose.

It is in these two ways—antibody assay of blood and skin testing—that allergy clinics will detect which offending agents are causing allergy. There is no controversy about the disease group, its causes, or the mechanisms involved. There are other tests used to detect more delayed types of allergic reaction, but these tests remain controversial, and the exact mechanisms of action are as yet unclear.

Such tests indicate that only 1% of the general population can be said to be truly allergic to a particular food. However, for children the figure has been estimated to be around 5%.

Many of these children will outgrow their allergy, and by the time they reach the age of three, half of those allergic to milk or eggs will no longer be so. Many people who suffer allergy-type symptoms after eating attribute them to allergy—but they are often wrong to do so. In a survey conducted in 1994 on the adult population of High Wycombe, England, 20% said they were allergic to one food or another. When these people were subjected to double blind tests it was found that only 1% were truly allergic, from which we can infer that the remaining 19% were experiencing intolerance symptoms. Those who ascribe the intolerance reactions to 'pseudo-allergy' are also wrong, as nothing akin to an allergy mechanism is involved. The illness is a clear result of poisoning by a toxin: in other words, food intolerance. Far more than 1% of people suffer from this—maybe 20%, one person in five—and as we have already seen with alcohol and MSG, those who have an inefficient detoxification system will suffer more than most.

So what are the other hidden dangers in our food? How do we spot them? The following chapters tell you.

CHAPTER 4

The biogenic amines

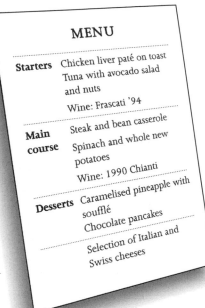

MENU

Starters Chicken liver paté on toast
Tuna with avocado salad
and nuts
Wine: Frascati '94

**Main
course** Steak and bean casserole
Spinach and whole new
potatoes
Wine: 1990 Chianti

Desserts Caramelised pineapple with
soufflé
Chocolate pancakes

Selection of Italian and
Swiss cheeses

This menu looks delicious; it is also well balanced and highly nutritious. But it contains foods that are naturally high in biogenic amines, which can give most people a headache. All that is required is about 100 mg of the biogenic amine—a mere tenth of a gram. Assuming the guests at a banquet ate normal sized portions, they would get more than twice this amount; and while this will not produce an *allergic* reaction, it will mean that they have more biogenic amine than can be removed rapidly from the body. The result is likely to be a throbbing headache lasting several hours. By themselves, the foods on this menu can be tolerated with no problems, but together they stimulate receptors and overload the body's mechanisms for detoxifying biogenic amines.

Biogenic amines are very active, and are involved in many of the vital functions of the body. They are needed all the time, as blood is being pumped, air is being breathed in and out, the brain is thinking, our limbs are moving, and our senses are operating. These, and a thousand other activities, are being driven by millions of chemical reactions. We are unaware of them, but body processes are continuously starting and stopping, accelerating and slowing down—and many are controlled by the biogenic amines.

The name 'biogenic' means 'biologically developed', and these chemicals are formed naturally within the body. They are also made by other animals and by plants, and so they are present in a wide range of foods. In the human body, biogenic amines act as neurotransmitters—in other words, they carry messages to receptors which are thereby triggered into action—and they have to be kept strictly under control: the body has powerful mechanisms for neutralising them once their job is done. But if there is just too much to cope with—for example, someone has eaten foods rich in biogenic amines—or if the person is ill and their defences are depleted, then the effects can be dramatic. Biogenic amines can stimulate the arteries, causing headaches. They may affect the central nervous system, causing sleepiness and fatigue, and restrict the air passages, resulting in wheezing. There may also be more muted responses, but the symptoms produced, such as diarrhoea, mood swings, nausea, and bloating, can be debilitating.

In this chapter we look more closely at what is happening when these reactions occur, but first we need to know more about the biogenic amines themselves.

Body receptors and naturally occurring amines

The biogenic amines that can provoke food intolerance are formed from amino acids by specific enzymes that can remove the acid group and leave the amino group. Many amines so formed have a valuable role to play as neurotransmitters governing various body processes. For example, the amines needed for the working of the brain are serotonin, melatonin, and dopamine. Serotonin will trigger receptors that control blood vessels so that they dilate or contract, according to the need for blood. If there is too much contraction in the brain, we experience a migraine. Serotonin also regulates the functions of the pituitary gland, which is the major hormone controller. Appetite, sleep, mood, and the perception of pain are likely to be affected if there is any interference with this neurotransmitter: depletion of serotonin leads to depression, insomnia, and over-eating, and the outcome may be obesity.

For medical reasons we may want to control our serotonin levels, and this we can do by taking drugs known as SRRIs (serotonin receptor re-uptake inhibitors) of which Prozac is the best known. On the other hand, we may want to experience the effects of extra serotonin, and there are drugs that will mimic the effects of serotonin and activate some of the receptors that are sensitive to it. Ecstasy is one such drug: it acts as a super-serotonin, and its effects will last several hours because the body can not remove it very quickly. It affects the brain's neurotransmitters, especially dopamine and noradrenaline, producing the 'rave' effect. The dopamine makes us feel good, but it is the noradrenaline that counteracts the effect of serotonin, making us energetic and wide awake, to the extent that we can dance happily all night. Ecstasy also raises body temperature, causing dehydration, and this leads to the major side-effect of heat exhaustion. Ecstasy was originally intended for suppressing appetite, which it can do by mimicking serotonin.

Once a biogenic amine has done its job, the body needs to be rid of it, so it detoxifies and excretes it. This is done using enzymes. The first enzyme, known as an monoamine oxidase, removes the amino group from the biogenic amine, and replaces it with an aldehyde group. This type of chemical is also highly reactive, and it too needs to be detoxified. We rely on another enzyme, called aldehyde dehydrogenase, to convert the aldehyde to an acid. These acids are readily soluble in water, and enter the bloodstream. Unless they can be used elsewhere in the body, they will be filtered out by the kidneys.

Occasionally there may be an excess of a biogenic amine in the food we eat. This is what happened in the case of Rosemary, as the box explains.

Case study: **What Rosemary ate at the health-food bistro**

Rosemary, a 48-year-old women, had lunch out with a friend, at a health food bistro. She had a tuna fish bake with a green salad, and a glass of white wine. She was in good spirits, and she chatted happily with her friend for an hour or so. They parted after the meal, but as Rosemary drove home she began to feel strange. She thought the glass of wine was affecting her as she felt slightly light-headed, a symptom that she recognised as indicating the start of a migraine. Then her palms started to itch, followed by the soles of her feet and her lips. Finally she was itching all over, and as she scratched her skin it produced red weals and flared.

She only just reached home before she was violently sick. This was followed by diarrhoea, and accompanied by colicky and severe abdominal pain, plus a thumping headache. This pattern continued for several hours, and if she attempted to stand up she felt very faint. Her husband rang the doctor and described her symptoms, and was surprised to be told that in 12 hours they would clear completely. Though Rosemary would feel washed out, she would suffer no serious after-effects. Things turned out just as the doctor said they would.

Rosemary was suffering a classic case of amine intolerance, which has very rapid onset which involves the whole body. The condition was not helped by the wine she had drunk, but the fish was the cause of her attack. The tuna she had eaten was probably not fresh tuna, nor from a newly opened can, but fish that had been stored in conditions that permitted enzymes to break down its amino acids to produce unacceptable levels of biogenic amine.

Table 4.1 lists the key biogenic amines, the amino acids from which they derive, and the foods that have high levels of these amino acids. These levels will increase in the case of fruit and vegetables as they ripen, and increase further as they start to spoil (with the exception of pineapple where the levels actually fall). Processing, canning, pickling, and juicing may also increase these levels, and most biogenic amines are heat-resistant. Most dangerous are foods that have begun to spoil. Then we see intolerance reactions that require urgent medical help.

The production of biogenic amine neurotransmitters in the body relies on the levels of the amino acid precursors from which they derive. So production can be increased by increasing the amount of the appropriate amino acids in the diet. For example, increasing tryptophan intake increases the level of serotonin. Conversely, some diets that are low in tryptophan cause the levels of this amine to drop, and this occurs in regions where corn, which is low in tryptophan, is the staple food, rather than wheat or rice.

While it is generally beneficial to have a diet rich in proteins, the supply of amino acids this provides may also give rise to free biogenic amines. The danger from these comes if the body can not easily deal with them, and this can happen to patients receiving monoamine oxidase inhibitor (MAOI) drugs, which defuse the enzyme that is involved in the first stage of detoxification.

Table 4.1 The biogenic amines and the foods in which they occur.

Biogenic amine	Amino acid from which it is derived	Foods with high levels of this amino acid	Foods that are likely to contain excess free amine
Histamine	histidine	eggs, herbs, cheese, potatoes, nuts, fish	yeast products (e.g. Marmite), blue cheese, Swiss cheese, tuna, salami, spinach, red wine
Serotonin (5-hydroxy-tryptamine)	tryptophan	fish, meat, herbs, diary products	chocolate, wines, pickled fish, cheese, banana, pineapple, avocado, plums, tomatoes, octopus
Dopamine	phenylalanine	grains, nuts, meat, fish, diary products, beans	banana, avocado
Tyramine	tyrosine	dairy foods, eggs, salmon, spinach, processed meats, nuts	oranges, plums, tomato, fruit juices
Tryptamine	tryptophan	grains, nuts, meat, fish, dairy products, beans	cheese, pickled herrings, sausages
Phenylethylamine	phenylalanine	grains, nuts, meat, fish, dairy products, beans	chocolate, cheese, salted and pickled fish, meat extracts, liver, sausages, wines, beer
Octopamine	tyrosine	dairy foods, eggs, salmon, spinach, processed meats, nuts	oranges, plums, tomato, fruit juices

A person needs to be in a balanced and responsive state to lead a normal life, and it was suggested many years ago that chronically depressed people might be deficient in histamine in their brain cells. One way of making more of this amine available was to block the enzyme that removes it, i.e. to reduce the amount of monoamine oxidase by treating them with an MAOI drug. Drugs of this kind have been used successfully for many years as anti-depressants in treating chronically sick, and clinically depressed, patients who are resistant to other forms of treatment. Some of these patients suffered a side-effect: if they ate certain cheeses, wines, and fish—all containing high levels of biogenic amines—then what looked like severe histamine poisoning would occur because the amine removal system had been blocked by the drugs, and was not functioning. The symptoms were increased blood pressure, tremors, convulsions, and, occasionally, death.

In 1963 it was suggested that the culprit was not actually histamine, but another biogenic amine—one that is not used by the body, but which stimulates the same receptors and utilises the same degradation pathways. This amine was called tyramine. In the same year A. M. Asatoor published in the *Lancet* the levels of tyramine occurring naturally in aged cheese, and suggested that it was capable of interacting with the blocked degradation pathways. Those on MAOI drugs showed a marked rise in blood pressure if they ate this type of cheese. Soon more foods were implicated, including beer, wine, pickled herrings, coffee, avocado, nuts, yeast, broad bean pods, chicken liver, and canned figs. It is now generally accepted that both histamine and tyramine exist in these foods and both can cause food intolerance.

Histamine

Histamine is one of the most common naturally occurring chemicals in the body, but it can be lethal, and the level of it has to be strictly controlled. It is also one of the most common hidden dangers in our diet, and can be found in a wide range of foods. We may be unaware of its presence in food that has been spoiled by bacteria: the damage may not be obvious enough to alert us to the danger, but may be sufficient to pose a threat.

The first time histamine poisoning was reported was in 1830, when five crew members on the vessel *Triton of Leith* complained of violent headaches, flushed skin, swollen faces, shivering, and diarrhoea. This had started after they had eaten the fish bonito. At the time this new illness was termed 'scombroid poisoning', after the Scomberesocidae, the family of fish most commonly associated with it, which includes mackerel, tuna, and bonito. The poisoning has also been reported with other fish, such as jacks, herrings, sardines, pilchards, and anchovies. But today we know that the illness is due to histamine, and the symptoms it causes have become well recognized.

Scombroid poisoning is most common in the USA, Japan, and Europe. In the UK there were 438 suspected cases in the years 1976–1990, and these involved 962 people of whom 167 were confirmed by analysis as having been poisoned by histamine. Histamine poisoning has an extremely rapid onset, and can start in as little as ten minutes, or take up to two hours. Usually it lasts about 12 hours and is evidenced by rashes, sweating, shivering, flushing, diarrhoea, a burning sensation in the mouth, and abdominal cramp. The case histories in the box show what can happen.

Two case studies: **On the menu, but off**

Case 1

A 45-year-old man began to feel unwell in the afternoon, soon after he returned to work after dining at a wine bar. Within a few hours he was so ill he went to see his doctor, by which time he exhibited symptoms of face and throat swelling, flushing, headache, and diarrhoea. The symptoms had started after he had eaten a large, grilled, supposedly fresh, tuna steak, and food poisoning was suspected. Happily his condition righted itself after a few hours, but an investigation of the cause was initiated. Of the three portions of tuna served to customers that day, two were known to have caused illness. Samples were taken from the same fish, and analysis showed levels of histamine in excess of 200 mg per 100 gram of fish, whereas the normal safe limit is 5 mg. Levels in excess of 50 mg are regarded as potentially toxic. Because the fresh tuna had been left standing in a warm room for too long before cooking, degradation of the fish had begun, and histamine had been released. Subsequent cooking arrested the decomposition, but did not destroy the histamine that had been produced.

Case 2

A 31-year-old man suddenly found a rash all over his face and upper body. His doctor confirmed that it had been caused by something he had recently eaten, and suspicion fell on some tuna and mayonnaise sandwiches. The cause was confirmed when six other staff in the office where he worked also became ill, with similar symptoms including headache, flushing, rash, and diarrhoea. They too had eaten the same sandwiches for lunch. All the symptoms disappeared within a few hours of onset. Samples of the tuna mayonnaise filling were obtained the same afternoon, and sent for analysis. They showed levels of histamine in excess of 250 mg per 100 g of filling. The can from which the tuna had been taken had been opened at about 6 a.m. that day, and the tuna had then been mixed with mayonnaise. However, this was then left to stand for several hours in a warm kitchen before being used to make sandwiches, and these were also not refrigerated before being sold.*

*Taken from Ian M. Stell, Trouble with tuna: two cases of scombrotoxin poisoning. *Journal of Accidental and Emergency Medicine*, 1997, Vol. 14, pp. 110–17.

The level of histamine in Scomberesocidae fish is usually less than 20 mg per 100 g, but spoilage results in the naturally occurring precursor, the amino acid histidine, breaking down to form the active agent histamine, under the action of the enzyme histidine decarboxylase. Bacteria that produce this enzyme are commonly found in the skin, gills, and gut of fish, and it becomes active if the fish is kept at temperatures higher than 4 °C. This is why it is essential for raw fish to be properly stored by refrigeration. Because histamine is heat stable, cooking the fish does not subsequently remove it, so histamine can be present and remain active after canning. This latter fact was reported in 1974 by Michael Merson and co-workers in the *Journal of the American Medical Association*, where they recorded a case in which 232 people had been poisoned by two lots of commercially canned tuna. The report makes interesting reading because it shows the variety and frequency of the symptoms of histamine poisoning, the time lapse between eating the suspect food and the onset of symptoms, and the levels of histamine in the contaminated and uncontaminated cans:

On February 20th 1973, US Food and Drug Administration (FDA) officials learned of an illness characterized by gastrointestinal symptoms, flushing, and headache in persons living in three north-central states. The illness was thought to be related to the consumption of commercially canned tuna fish. Preliminary investigation by the FDA and the Center for Disease Control (CDC) confirmed that about 150 cases of ... scombroid fish poisoning had occurred after the consumption of tuna fish from two lots produced by one canner.

On February 23rd, the canner recalled the 170,000 cans in the two lots, and the FDA issued a nationwide press release advising against the eating of the contaminated fish and asking that cans from the implicated lots be returned.... Three days later, a telephone survey of all state health departments was conducted.

Four state health departments confirmed 232 cases. Symptoms of 95 patients interviewed included nausea (86%), cramps (71%), oral blistering or burning sensation (63%), diarrhoea

(55%), flushing (46%), rash including urticaria (32%) and vomiting (27%). Palpitations were also reported. Although some persons who were affected consulted their physicians no case required hospitalization, and no deaths were reported. The mean of the reported incubation periods was approximately 45 minutes, with a range of 15 minutes to three hours. The duration of the illness was generally eight hours or less.

On February 25th, FDA laboratories reported that nine assays of fish from the incriminated lots showed 68 to 280 mg of histamine per 100 grams of fish; seven of the nine assays showed 180 mg per 100 gram or higher. Assays of histamine in three samples of tuna from another company revealed an average concentration of 3 mg per 100 grams.

Food contaminated with histamine can deliver enough to swamp the body's defences. Yet the cells of the body already contain enough histamine to do this, which is why it has to be securely held in check. This histamine is stored in an inert state, as granules, which can be transported around the body safely. In this way the histamine can be supplied to the right place, at right time, and in the right quantities, to produce the effects which the body seeks. Like all neurotransmitters, it has to be assembled from its precursors, in this case the amino acid histidine. The inert granules release the active histamine in a process called degranulation.

If something interferes with this process, we can poison ourselves with an overdose of histamine from within our own bodies. For example, various chemicals cause degranulation, releasing histamine from its controlled state so that it becomes free and active. This can trigger a whole series of symptoms. Two important agents in food that will do this are metabisulfites, a chemical used in the brewing and food industries to stop rogue yeasts causing fermentation, and salicylates, a natural chemical related to aspirin. Chapters 5 and 6 deal with these hidden dangers.

Sir Henry Dale and his colleagues at the end of the nineteenth century were working on derivatives of the ergot alkaloids when they first isolated histamine. They observed its potent action on smooth muscle in the capillary blood vessels, and noted the similarity with the acute allergic reaction known as anaphylactic shock. They also demonstrated that histamine was released from the lung during anaphylactic shock, where it not only affected blood vessels, but it also constricted the air passages known as the bronchioles. Other workers showed histamine to be present in a whole range of different tissues, and it was slowly realised that histamine was exerting its influence by stimulating specific receptors in the body.

Pharmaceutical companies began to produce antihistamines, drugs that were specifically antagonistic to histamine, but the early ones did not appear to block all the effects: for example, histamine causes stomach juices to flow, but the antihistamines did not stop them. In the 1960s, however, a second type of histamine receptor was identified, and this was labelled H_2 to distinguish it from the first type, which were now called H_1 receptors. Both were responsive to histamine, but resulted in two quite distinct sets of actions.

By the 1970s specific H_2 antagonists had been developed, and this led to important new treatments for stomach ulceration—within a few years the need for surgery in this debilitating illness had all but disappeared. Ulcers are caused by damage to the stomach wall—initially due to alcohol, smoking, or *Heliobacter pylori* bacteria—which is then unable to heal because of the high acidity. Histamine promotes the flow of acid, so if this is controlled by blocking the H_2 receptors then the ulcer will generally heal within a few days.

In the 1960s a general surgical ward of any hospital would have had a large proportion of its patients waiting for, or recovering from, gastric surgery to remove ulcers. This would be done by cutting the nerves to the stomach and refashioning it to enable it to empty more quickly. Alternatively, the acid-generating part of the stomach would be cut out. These were major operations and invalided the patient for weeks. Nor was the operation always success-ful, and further surgery was sometimes required, even to the extent of total removal of the stomach. But in the early 1970s James Black, working at Smith Kline Beecham, found that the H_2 receptors could be blocked, and the chemicals that produced this effect were modified until a safe form was found. This was the drug cimetidine, and, along with others that were to follow, it revolutionised the treatment of stomach ulcers. Today, you would be unlikely to find any patient on a surgical ward who was waiting for such an operation on a gastric ulcer.

Finally, in the 1980s, a third type of histamine-activated receptor was identified, and called H_3. This had specific actions in brain tissues and consequently influenced brain activ-ity, such as sleep, appetite, and alertness. We should no longer be surprised that, having three different receptors to activate, histamine can produce such a wide range of symptoms when it is massively released in the body, or is taken in with our food.

Wines can trigger histamine release in the body, but some wines such as sherry also con-tain high levels of histamine. Attempts to reduce these levels have not always met with suc-cess. For example, in April 1997 a new type of sherry was announced which would not cause a hangover: Jose Estevez, of Jerez, had produced a pale dry Tio Mateo that contained prac-tically no histamine. He had bought two sherry bodegas that had fallen on hard times, and had invested a great deal of his time and money in trying to find a way to revive them in the face of a declining market for sherry. This once-popular aperitif had gained a reputation for causing headaches, so Estevez decided to produce a healthier, low-histamine wine. He teamed up with the German firm Underberg, which made a low-histamine sparkling wine, and had a laboratory in Switzerland. The formation of histamine in the sherry was con-trolled by using a kind of yeast that helped the sherry ferment, and by ensuring that rogue yeasts didn't infect the grape juice.

To begin with, the response to Estevez's sherry was favourable. The Spanish chairman of the European Histamine Research Society, Felix Lopez Elorza, gave it his approval: 'Wine with less histamine is definitely healthier, especially for people who have difficulty eliminat-ing histamine, which is possibly from about 4–7% of the population.' Support for the new type of sherry also came from Francisco Bravo, a research professor of chemistry and oenol-ogy (the study of wines) at Madrid's Center for Scientific Studies. He was quoted as saying: 'Low-histamine wine has great value from a medical point of view, especially for those who must reduce the amount of histamine in their diet. It is a toxic substance, especially in combination with the alcohol in wine.'

Sadly, the new sherry could not be labelled as 'low-histamine' because this is forbidden by Spanish law and was opposed by the sherry-makers. The ruling was supported by the Federation of Sherry Exporters, who maintain that histamine is a natural product formed in the fermentation process, and that the body has a natural defence mechanism to cope with it. This, as we have seen, is true—provided the amount is small. For those who are sensitive to too much histamine, then sherry must remain a drink to avoid, despite Jose Estevez's brave attempts to make it safe.

Serotonin (5-hydroxytryptamine)

Serotonin is the more common name for the amine 5-hydroxytryptamine. It is one of our most important neurotransmitters, and is linked very closely with mood, appetite, sex, and sleep. These four actions do not just occur at random: they are triggered by the activation of specific nervous receptors. For example, when the receptors governing sleep are stimulated by serotonin, tiredness ensues, and the individual then falls asleep. The sleep deepens through various levels, until rapid eye movement (REM) occurs. This is the most important kind of sleep, during which the brain organises the information it has collected during the day. Because all the newer types of anti-depressants work by controlling serotonin, there can be an unwanted side effect in about 10% of patients: they put on weight.

Appetite is also influenced by serotonin and much research has been published on the drugs that affect this relationship. One such, dexfenfluramine, blocks the serotonin and delays emptying of the stomach after a solid meal. It thereby decreases the appetite, although it does not work with a liquid diet. Other workers showed that the same drug acted centrally in the brain, altering the release of corticosteroid hormones, which in turn can affect body weight.

Serotonin is present at high levels in platelets in the blood. It is held in an inert state, but on release it is thought to be involved in blood clotting and inflammation. Its importance in this role has been known for over a century, and it was viewed as a nuisance in laboratories where this powerful agent would cause blood vessels to constrict, often ruining an experiment. The name serotonin was coined in 1949, from 'sero', meaning of the blood, and 'tonin', which refers to the contractile properties that the chemical possesses. This new chemical was identified and finally synthesised two years later. So much work on serotonin followed, that within two years there were more than 4000 references to it in the scientific literature.

There are also large quantities of serotonin in the brain, and one theory links reduced levels to certain mental conditions such as depression. The most recent drugs used to treat depression inhibit serotonin re-uptake at receptors. Research continues as to how it is depleted, and whether it can enhance mood if more is made available. It may be possible to encourage its manufacture in the body, or to block the route by which it is degraded. Either way, higher levels of serotonin should lead to mood elevation. Some researchers have suggested that a diet low in tryptophan, the amino acid from which it is derived, can cause depression, and they advocate restoring tryptophan levels by dietary means as a way of successfully treating the condition. But this theory remains conjecture, and clearly other interactions and processes play a part.

The ban on over-the-counter sales of tryptophan that was imposed by the FDA in 1989 followed the deaths of 30 people who used this amino acid as a dietary supplement. The agent responsible for causing the rare illness that killed them, sinophalia-myalgria syndrome, was tracked to oxidised forms of tryptophan in the contaminated product.

Case study: **The meat-and-two-veg man**

Roy, at 52, is the headmaster of a large school. He was troubled by regular migraine attacks once or twice a month, but more troublesome was severe stiffness in his joints in the morning, which in some instances would last for several days. He had been thoroughly investigated medically, but no underlying cause had been found. It was suggested that something in his diet might be to blame.

The first action taken by the clinic to which Roy was referred was to collect data about all the food he ate over the following two weeks. In such a survey the patient is given a list of foods and the option to score them as: never, occasionally, or regularly eaten, the latter accompanied by careful assessment of the size of all the portions that have been consumed. Standard allergy testing, in combination with the questionnaire, formed the basis of the analysis, but it was immediately apparent Roy was a traditional meat-and-two-veg man, with the emphasis on the meat. He ate a great deal of beef, lamb, and pork.

His dietary survey confirmed this, and on questioning Roy admitted to eating very little fish, poultry, or dairy products. He was persuaded to change his diet for a month, adding one or two other foods, such as turkey, duck, or fish. At the same time, he increased the ratio of vegetables to meat. Soon he began to feel better, and six months later he was free of joint pains, although he still had occasional migraines. He had identified by trial and error that beef and lamb were to the meats to avoid; pork did not seem to bring on any symptoms.

There was no evidence that Roy was allergic to anything, and his was a simple case of free amine overload due to a diet rich in tryptophan. The amine most implicated was serotonin. All meats have serotonin, but levels vary; a diet consistently high in a particular meat can result in a high intake of serotonin.

Too much tryptophan-rich protein may lead to an excess of serotonin that can upset the body in different ways, as the case study in the box shows.

Vitamin B_6 is needed to generate neurotransmitters from tryptophan, and if this vitamin is lacking, or has been destroyed by cooking, then these neurotransmitters will be depleted. An example is given in Chapter 10 of a case in which this vitamin was lacking in formula feeds for babies. A similar situation occurs in some women who take oral contraceptives, which interfere with neurotransmitter production. They become depressed, and this depression often lifts dramatically when extra vitamin B_6 supplements are taken.

Free serotonin is found in a number of foods, and especially in those such as pineapples, bananas, plums, avocados, and tomatoes which lend themselves to processing into juices, concentrates, pulps, purees and preserves. Such processing leads to higher concentrations of this biogenic amine.

The body has a very efficient neutralising system for free serotonin, using oxidases and methyl transferase. Evidence of these neutralising mechanisms is to be found in the breakdown products that occur in the spinal fluids, blood, and urine.

At one stage in its detoxification, serotonin competes for the same enzyme that is needed to remove the acetaldehyde that is produced in the detoxification of alcohol, as described in Chapter 2. Since there is so much acetaldehyde to be removed compared to the amount of serotonin, there is a build-up of this neurotransmitter in the brain, and this may explain some of the mental changes that happen when we have had a lot to drink.

Some people, like Roy the headmaster, suffer joint pains after eating certain foods. Where there is definite evidence of joint inflammation, but no evidence of rheumatoid arthritis or osteoarthritis as its cause, serotonin may be to blame. Tests can reveal whether serotonin levels are raised in the blood, and its breakdown products can be detected in the urine. These tests are carried out after the patient has been 'challenged' with the offending foods under experimental conditions. In Roy's case his restricted diet, nutritious though it was in all other respects, guaranteed him more free serotonin than his enzyme system could deal with.

A serotonin-related mechanism has also been suggested for migraine. The release of serotonin in the blood starts a chain reaction affecting both nerve endings and the blood vessels in the brain. This results in the vascular/pulsatile type of headache typical of migraine. The levels of breakdown products excreted in the urine once again record the extent of serotonin release. Those who suffer from inexplicable migraine might well experiment with their diet and cut out foods that contain above-average amounts of serotonin, as shown in Table 4.1.

Dopamine and phenylethylamine

Dopamine and phenylethylamine have been closely associated in the scientific literature with changes in mood, behaviour, and co-ordination. Dopamine is an important neurotransmitter in the brain, and phenylethylamine is produced from it. Whether phenylethylamine can also affect the brain is uncertain, because it is not capable of acting as a neurotransmitter; but it is a false transmitter and as such it has similarities to other molecules, such as amphetamines, that are physiologically active. However, there is no evidence that the body treats phenylethylamine as anything other than a chemical to be removed.

Phenylethylamine is found in a number of foods, particularly chocolate, Gouda and Stilton cheeses, sausages, meat extracts, red wine, and certain pickled foods. Studies have been undertaken on people who believed their migraines and headaches were due to chocolate, and these established that there was a relationship between the headache and the phenylethylamine in the chocolate. Such people do not have sufficient of the enzyme that breaks phenylethylamine down.

Chocolate is one of the foods that commonly induces bingeing, the inability to control one's eating. Bouts of uncontrolled eating are followed by induced vomiting and further frenetic eating. Loss of appetite, bingeing, anorexia, and the bulimic syndromes have received a great deal of attention from research workers, and many animal models have been designed to investigate the biochemistry. It is thought that bingeing may be the result of a central nervous system abnormality, where the appetite mechanism is interfered with by phenylethylamine. The levels of dopamine set free from cells and the levels of phenylethylamine that result are linked in a complex of interactions that are not yet fully understood. These compounds control a number of 'pleasure' centres in the brain, one of which concerns the satisfaction of feeling full after a meal, which is the normal cue to stop eating. So it is likely that both anorexia, and overeating leading to obesity, involve these biogenic amines, dopamine and phenylethylamine.

Case study: **The chocolate kid**

Andrew, aged 12, went to boarding school, where his teachers found him difficult to deal with because of his attention deficit and intermittent unruly behaviour. With the agreement of his parents he was referred to an allergy clinic.

Andrew arrived at the clinic overweight, flushed, and with his pockets bulging. He paid little attention to the questions asked by the doctor. He was asked to empty his pockets, and this revealed three different types of chocolate bar and a packet of chewy fruit sweets. Rather than eat the school meals, which he did only selectively, he used the school shop for the majority of his diet and would eat anything up to six chocolate bars per day. Reluctantly, Andrew agreed that for two weeks he would eat school meals and avoid all chocolate, replacing it with fruit of his choice.

The school rang the clinic three days later, saying that Andrew's behaviour was even worse than usual, but they were urged to persevere with the new regime. It paid off: two weeks later, when Andrew again visited the clinic, he sat quietly and attentively. Not surprisingly, he had lost weight. His teachers had noted an improvement in his behaviour, but whether this was the introduction of a sensible diet, or the elimination of chocolate, was debatable. Following closer analysis it was concluded that phenylethylamine and dopamine has been at the bottom of Andrew's earlier problems of aggressive behaviour and inability to concentrate. When he was again allowed to eat excess chocolate, his bad behaviour pattern re-emerged.

Raised levels of phenylethylamine in blood occur in patients with schizophrenia, and several researchers have suggested there may be a link between them. Support for this theory comes from the fact that noradrenalin and adrenalin, the parent compounds that produce dopamine and phenylethylamine, have a role in so many of the body's vital functions. Though no direct causal effect has been demonstrated in schizophrenia, tests show that abnormal amounts of dopamine are produced when its precursor molecule, phenylalanine, has been ingested. Like all these rather tenuous associations the results need cautious assessment, but when linked to the other types of amine problems it seems likely that dietary causes are involved.

Dopamine is perhaps best known for its association with Parkinson's disease. In this disease the patient experiences a tremor that markedly increases with age. Examination of patients shows that the area of the brain concerned with co-ordination is low in dopamine, but it can not be replenished from the diet because of the systems that stop the transport of dopamine into the brain.

Parkinson's disease is named after a London doctor, James Parkinson. In 1817 he wrote an article entitled 'An essay on the shaking palsy', which described the symptoms of a curious ailment that afflicted people in old age. In the last century nothing could be done to halt its remorseless progress, which eventually left its victim unable to perform even the simplest everyday action. In addition to the obvious tremor, the body became bent at the knees and hips, and speech and swallowing were difficult. Yet there was no loss of mental capacity, as we know from Alexander von Humbolt (1769–1859), the German naturalist and chemist, who had the disease and kept a record of its progression.

About 10 000 new cases of Parkinson's disease are diagnosed in the UK each year, and the numbers are growing as the population ages. The incidence of the disease is only 80 per million in people younger than 50, but this rises to 22 000 per million of those over 70. It is not a hereditary disease, and it appears to strike at random.

The discovery was made in the 1950s that Parkinson's disease was linked to the lack of dopamine, but injecting dopamine was not an effective treatment because it is broken down in the body before it can reach the brain. However, a related substance, levodopa, could be given, and this is converted to dopamine in the body by the enzyme dopadecarboxylase. The result is that a small amount of dopamine can penetrate through to the brain cells that are being starved of this neurotransmitter.

Although the body needs dopamine, it also wants to be rid of it after it has completed its role as a chemical messenger. We use two enzymes, monoamine oxidase (MAO) and catechol-O-methyl transferase (COMT), to do this, and while the dopamine-producing cells gradually disappear with age, the ability to remove dopamine does not. However, a normal person can function perfectly adequately with only 30% of his or her dopamine neurones working: but fall below this, and symptoms of the disease appear. Drugs that inhibit MAO and COMT allow people with Parkinson's disease to make the most of their dwindling supply of dopamine. Selegiline, which was introduced in the early 1970s, inhibits MAO, and so enables more dopamine to remain active. Similarly, tolcapone and entacapone drugs inhibit the COMT enzyme, and these were launched in 1997 and 1998. Ropinrole was launched in 1996, and this is a dopamine agonist—in other words, it can act in place of dopamine at the chemical messenger sites that dopamine should be targeting. The drug pramipexole works in the same way.

Tyramine and octopamine

In addition to the useful neurotransmitters that occasionally go astray, there are also the false neurotransmitters that serve no useful purpose. Tyramine and octopamine come into this category. Though neither is as active as the genuine neurotransmitters, they can fool the receptors and lock on to them, so preventing the useful ones attaching themselves, and thereby preventing the correct instructions from being sent out. While tyramine has no natural function in the body, it has been put to use in medical research a means of displacing noradrenalin at nerve endings.

Many foods contain small amounts of tyramine and octopamine, and some foods contain large amounts. The wine Chianti has particularly high levels of tyramine, as do cheeses such as Camembert and Stilton. While most people can cope with a moderate intake of tyramine and octopamine, when they are exposed to foods such as these, they experience an intolerance reaction that often takes the form of migraine attacks. This happens because tyramine is also vasoactive: it affects blood vessels, leading to increased blood pressure, and causes migraine not just in susceptible individuals, but in most people. Studies on volunteers have shown that 100–125 mg of this biogenic amine will produce a severe headache in 90% of people.

Bacteria that spoil food, and those living naturally in the gut, produce enzymes that work on the amino acid tyrosine, which is found in some foods when they are going off. The enzymes turn the tyrosine into tyramine and then into octopamine, both of which provoke a toxic response in the form of headaches, sleepiness, and mood change. This is why the level of tyramine in food can depend on how it is ripened, fermented, cooked, or stored.

Case study: Family dinners became a real pain

Jackie is a 48-year-old woman who had frequent migraine attacks accompanied by visual disturbances that took the form of zigzag flashes, a pulsating headache, nausea, and vomiting. Attacks occurred three or four times a month. She noticed that they were particularly likely to occur after the weekend, and in her opinion it was probably red wine that was at fault. She drank this when her family came round for a roast meal on Sundays. Avoiding red wine, however, did not prevent the attacks.

Jackie consulted her doctor who advised her to attend an allergy clinic, where she was found to be sensitive to potato. When challenged with this vegetable she did have a mild migraine attack, and blood tests showed a positive antibody response to potato and to several other foods, including tomato, chicken, beef, and broccoli.

After eliminating these from her diet for several weeks she noticed a decrease in the frequency and severity of attacks, but headaches still occurred quite regularly, and something else was clearly to blame. Attention finally focused on tyramine as the most likely agent responsible. Jackie was given a list of all foods containing this amine, which she then avoided. As a result she had no more headaches, and had only one migraine attack in the next nine months.

Table A2.1 in Appendix 2 lists tyramine-containing foods, and Table 4.2 includes a few foods that have particularly high levels of this biogenic amine. There are other foods that are rich in tyramine, such as fermented sausages, sour cream, raspberries, and certain wines, and several where the amount depends on the food's freshness, and where spoilage can lead to high levels.

Although tyramine and octopamine are usually produced by bacteria, our own gut can sometimes generate them, especially in severe illness such as hepatic coma. High levels, from whatever source, have a profound effect, as will low levels for those taking MAOI drugs. Researchers studying such patients found that they react to tyramine at much lower doses than do other people, and observed that 10–25 mg would produce a severe reaction and 6–10 mg a mild reaction. Even foods containing very small amounts of tyramine can become a risk for these patients if enough is consumed, or if the foods are beginning to

Table 4.2 Foods containing high levels of tyramine.*

Food products	Tyramine content (mg per 100 g)
Camembert	up to 200
Emmental	20–100
Blue or Roquefort	up to 100
Gouda	up to 70
Boursault	10–110
Swiss	up to 180
Blue Stilton	50–230
Yeast extracts	up to 230
Pickled herrings	300
Sausages	up to 120

*For complete listing, see Table A2.1, pp. 168–9.

spoil. Symptoms can include a severe headache, usually at the back or side of the head, running eyes, salivation, and palpitations. Some people have even had heart attacks or stroke due to tyramine and octopamine. (Such reactions, however, are likely to result from the consumption of spoiled food, when levels of tyramine are much higher.) Clearly it is important to know which foods are to be avoided.

More than 200 foods contain tyramine in small quantities and have been implicated in adverse reactions in those undergoing MAOI treatment. Table A2.1 in Appendix 2, which lists some of these foods, was compiled by Stephen Sakland, Head of Pharmacy at the University of Texas, as a guide for those who are on such therapy.

Although we would be ill-advised to try to avoid all exposure to tyramine, it is possible to eat foods that contain very little. If you suspect that you react badly to this biogenic amine, you might experiment by excluding it from you diet for a while. This is not difficult, and the following foods can be eaten without worry, provided they are fresh.

anchovies	cream cheese	raisins
beetroot	cucumbers	salad dressings
chips (fries)	egg, boiled	sweet corn
colas	fish	tomato juice
coffee	mushrooms	yeast-leavened bread
cottage cheese	pineapple	

Dietary advice regarding biogenic amines

The foregoing advice on biogenic amines may be useful for people who are particularly susceptible to them. But there are a few general guidelines we can all follow if we want to reduce our exposure to foods that might be high in biogenic amines.

Alcoholic beverages Avoid red wine, and especially Chianti and vermouth, but a single glass (125 ml) of any wine, including these and port wine, presents little risk. Whisky, and liqueurs such as Drambuie and Chartreuse, can cause reactions. Beer should also be avoided, but some brands of beer are safe in small quantities. Some non-alcoholic beverages (alcohol-free beer and wines) may contain tyramine, and should be treated with caution.

Bean curd Fermented bean curd is often a part of Chinese and Japanese recipes, such as miso soup. This, and fermented soya bean and soya bean pastes, contain significant amounts of tyramine.

Cheese The tyramine content of cheese can not be predicted on the basis of its appearance, flavour, or variety, and therefore all cheeses should be avoided. However, exceptions are cream cheese and cottage cheese, which have no detectable levels of tyramine. This biogenic amine is the by-product of fermentation and aging, and so there is more in the more mature cheeses.

Fish and sea-food Fresh fish and vacuum-packed pickled fish contain only small amounts of tyramine, and are safe if they are consumed promptly or refrigerated for short periods; longer storage may be dangerous. Smoked, fermented, pickled, and otherwise aged fish should be avoided—pickled herrings especially so. Shrimp paste contains a large amount of tyramine.

Meat and meat products Fresh meat is safe, but processed meats may not be. Sausage, bologna, pepperoni, and salami are fermented, and contain large amounts of tyramine. No detectable tyramine levels are found in farm-cured ham. While tyramine is not found in fresh chicken livers, spoiled or old livers contain a lot. Meat extracts, and all liquid and powdered protein dietary supplements, should be avoided.

Sauerkraut The tyramine content of sauerkraut can be quite high.

Soups Soups generally should be avoided because they may contain protein extracts.

Yeast Neither brewer's yeast, nor yeast extracts (such as Vegemite or Marmite), nor yeast-based vitamin supplements should be consumed. Yeast in baking is safe.

The above is a list of foods to use with caution: it covers foods reported to cause hypertensive crisis (very high blood pressure) when they have been consumed in large quantities, stored for prolonged periods, or are contaminated. Small amounts of the following foods are not expected to pose a risk to those on MAOI therapy, although they may contain a little tyramine:

Avocados Do not eat avocados when they are over-ripe.

Chocolate Chocolate is safe, unless consumed in large amounts.

Dairy products Cream, sour cream, cottage cheese, cream cheese, yoghurt, and milk should pose little risk unless they have been stored for a long time or exposed to unhygienic conditions. Such products should not be used if they are near their sell-by or expiry date.

Nuts Nuts can generally be eaten, but avoid eating a lot of peanuts.

Raspberries Raspberries contain tyramine, so should only be eaten in small portions.

Spinach New Zealand spinach and hot weather spinach contain large amounts of tyramine. Other kinds of spinach do not.

Any protein food, improperly stored or handled, can form biogenic amines through protein breakdown. Chicken and beef liver, and liver pate, contain high amine levels, as does game which is hung to allow it to partially decompose as part of its preparation. Those on MAOI drugs should eat only fresh foods, and so long as these are purchased from reputable shops and stored properly, the danger of hypertensive (high blood pressure) crisis is minimal. Some foods should be avoided, the most dangerous being aged cheeses and yeast products used as food supplements.

At the start of this chapter we gave the menu of a meal high in biogenic amines, and if you look at it now you will see why it would leave some of the diners in a rather distressed state. Here instead is a typical menu which will cause much less agony from biogenic amines.

MENU

Starter	Fruit salad of fresh melon, grapes and pineapple
Main course	Roast duck with new potatoes, braised celery and runner beans
Dessert	Crème caramel
	Coffee

CHAPTER 5

Salicylates

```
                 MENU

Starter    Spicy salsa dip
           with crudities

Main       Tagliatelle Verde with
courses    tomato and oregano sauce
           Curried kofta balls with a
           yoghurt and tarragon sauce
           Ratatouille with broad beans
           All served with endive
           and chicory side salad

           Champagne

Dessert    Tropical fruit salad
           (pineapple, melon
           and mango)

           Special reserve port
```

This menu has been deliberately chosen for its high level of the non-nutrient salicylate, which can produce an intolerance response in some people. This is perhaps not surprising, because salicylate has a powerful effect on certain key enzymes in our body. Despite this, or because of it, many people deliberately take a daily dose of salicylate that is far in excess of what they would get if they chose from the above menu, and they do this in the form of an aspirin tablet. Aspirin is one form of salicylate: its chemical name is acetylsalicylic acid. Millions of people around the world take this common medicine in relatively large doses to relieve the minor aches and pains of life. Aspirin also reduces the incidence of coronary thrombosis and stroke, especially in patients who have a history of these conditions. It works by stopping the blood platelets clumping together and forming a clot, and is prescribed in 75 mg doses (junior aspirin size tablets). For pain relief the dose is much higher, at 4 g per day.

Salicylate, more than any of the other non-nutrients, produces a range of effects stretching from death, if a bottle of aspirin tablets is consumed, to the life-saving effects of aspirin taken as a prescribed medicine. Between these two we may experience a variety of responses to the drug, depending on how much we take and how sensitive we are to it. They may include serious side-effects, such as internal bleeding or mild poisoning, if we take a few too many tablets; or intolerance, if we are particularly sensitive to salicylate. But the vast majority of people get the response they seek, and for many it relieves their aches and pains.

For the few people who are ultra-sensitive to salicylate, there are salicylate-free diets. These regimes are almost impossible to follow without the help of a trained dietitian, because many food plants contain salicylate. A few foods contain no salicylate at all, and lots contain only tiny amounts, so it is possible to eat an *almost* salicylate free diet. In this chapter we will look first at the adverse effects salicylate may bring, and then at its dietary implications; and finally we will take a closer look at the actual benefits provided by a moderate intake of this non-nutrient.

Case study: **Roger, the athlete**

Roger (36 years old) is a top athlete and both a world and Olympic champion in his chosen sport. He suffered from colitis, a bowel disorder, which on one occasion clearly affected his performance. On some days, Roger said, he was lethargic and tired, and often had a severe headache. Training on those days was quite an effort. At such times he was depressed, he complained that his quality of life was poor, and he felt unable to cope.

When he discussed his eating habits, it became clear that Roger had quite a limited diet. He tended to eat lots of fruit and vegetables, and he liked pasta dishes with lots of sauce. Some meals definitely left him fatigued about an hour after he had eaten, but there was no allergic reaction or acute sensitivity to the food he was eating. He agreed to keep a detailed record of all his meals for two weeks, and to have a blood test. The analysis of his eating pattern showed a diet relatively high in salicylate, sometimes as much as 500 mg a day (which would be enough to cure a headache), and the blood test revealed that his white blood cells were reacting to this non-nutrient.

Roger was placed on a low salicylate diet, and he agreed, where possible, to substitute foods low in salicylate for those he had previously preferred. He had to give up pasta dishes, tomato sauces, baked beans, and vegetable curries. The annoying symptoms, including the bowel disorder, began to decline, and after a month they were no longer interfering with his training or life-style. As well as feeling better, Roger also noticed that his sporting performance was improving.

What is salicylate and what does it do?

Salicylates are the salts of salicylic acid (see the Glossary). The only common source of salicylate that we can overdose on, to the extent that it could threaten our life, is aspirin.

The acute lethal single dose of salicylate is about 20 g, which is equivalent to taking 40 adult-size aspirin tablets (500 mg each). As little as 4 g of aspirin may be fatal for a child—only eight of these tablets—which is why parents of young children should think twice before having a bottle of aspirin in the home. Another source of salicylate in the home is teething gel, which is rubbed on a baby's gums to reduce the discomfort of cutting its first teeth. This gel may well be based on oil of wintergreen, which is methyl salicylate, and this has been known to cause salicylate poisoning in young children who have eaten a whole tube of the gel.

There is a large amount of toxicological data about salicylate poisoning, sadly because an overdose of aspirin has often been used as a way of attempting suicide. As a result of treating people who have poisoned themselves this way, a lot is known about the effects that too much salicylate can have on the human body. The toxic effects are:

- rapid and deep breathing due to respiratory alkalosis, which is an abnormal shift in the acid–base balance of the body;
- reduction in bicarbonate levels in the blood, which upsets the sodium and potassium balance;
- dehydration and hypokalaemia, leading to coma;
- breakdown of normal cell metabolism;
- vital organ damage, mainly to the liver and kidneys, leading to death.

Poisoning by salicylate is a combination of disturbing the body's acid–base balance, and interfering with the process of oxidative phosphorylation, which is vital to the working of cells. The blood and tissue become too acidic, and essential minerals are unable to function correctly. At the same time, the body can not make the chemicals it needs to manufacture the high energy phosphates that enable it to draw on its main energy source, which is glucose.

As with any toxin, smaller doses produce milder upsets, from which the body can recover. But in a few susceptible people, even low levels of salicylates may induce intolerance symptoms. This can make life unpleasant, as they include urticaria (also known as nettle-rash or hives), swollen lips, swollen tongue, and difficulty in breathing, along with the more general symptoms of upset stomach, irregular bowel functions, and a general run-down feeling. For some people the response is immediate, even with relatively small amounts of aspirin, and they may suffer asthma, a blocked nose, or itching. This is similar to the effect of histamine, but it is not an allergic response. The greatest danger from aspirin is unseen: its effect on the gut wall. Some people experience this as indigestion, but others suffer catastrophic internal bleeding.

Despite these drawbacks, which affect only a few people, there are enormous benefits to be gained through taking aspirin. Most people can tolerate salicylate, and if they take a gram of aspirin (two tablets) every four hours, the effects can be beneficial in four ways: the salicylate acts as a painkiller; it lowers temperature; it combats inflammation; and it stimulates breathing. Doctors may prescribe aspirin as part of medical treatment, and then they rely on the following benefits to their patients: it controls blood sugar (glucose) and helps to remove uric acid, the chemical that causes gout; it prevents blood from clotting by decreasing the stickiness of platelets; and it reduces the risk of permanent damage in heart attacks and strokes.

Doctors are well aware that for some people there is a danger of internal bleeding, particularly in the stomach, and that aspirin is especially to be avoided in patients with a history of stomach ulcers. Even so, about two thirds of those who take an aspirin tablet experience a small amount of blood loss in the gut as a consequence, and this is thought to be worse in those who are deficient in vitamin C. Research done in the 1960s showed that one millilitre of blood is lost for every aspirin tablet taken. This is equivalent to a teaspoon-ful (5 ml) of blood if you take the usual eight tablets over two days that is normal in order to combat a cold.

Salicylates in food

In the 1970s doctors noticed that the symptoms of a mysterious 'disease X' were like those of patients who were taking aspirin and suffering its side-effects. The conclusion was that disease X was caused by salicylate from a different source: the diet. So began detailed inves-tigations into the salicylate content of food, and some surprising results were revealed by the careful work of Anne Swain, Stephen Dutton, and Stewart Truswell of the Human Nutrition Unit of the University of Sydney, Australia.

There are meals, like the one on the menu at the start of this chapter, that could provide enough salicylate to trigger a toxic response in anyone who was intolerant of this chemical. Herbs and spices are particularly high in salicylates, as Table 5.1 shows. Among the herbs, the highest levels are found in dill, mace, oregano, rosemary, tarragon, and thyme, while among the spices most salicylate is to be found in aniseed, cumin, curry powder, paprika, and turmeric. While some of these, such as curry powder and paprika, have remarkably large amounts, a meal made with them would have relatively little salicylate because a recipe needs only small amounts of these ingredients to achieve the desired flavour. For example, a heaped teaspoon of curry powder could provide 15 mg of salicylate.

Fruits have the highest levels of salicylate, as Table 5.2 shows. This table lists a repre-sentative selection of common foods; a more comprehensive list is given in Appendix 2, Table A2.2. Salicylate is produced by plants, and it concentrates in the surface layer of fruits and vegetables. Levels decrease as the fruit ripens. Green apples like Granny Smiths have a lot of salicylate, but Golden Delicious and Red Delicious varieties have rather less. Potatoes

Table 5.1 Herbs and spices.

Herbs	Salicylate*	Spices	Salicylate*
Bay leaf	2.52	Cardamom	7.7
Basil	3.4	Caraway	2.82
Coriander (fresh)	0.02	Cayenne	17.6
Dill	94.4	Chilli	1.30
Mace	32.2	Cinnamon	15.2
Mint	9.4	Cloves	5.74
Oregano	66	Cumin	45.0
Rosemary	68	Curry	218
Sage	21.7	Mustard	26
Tarragon	34.8	Paprika	203
Thyme	183	Pepper, black	6.2
Garlic, fresh clove	0.10	Turmeric	76.4

*milligrams per 100 g of the dried or powdered form, except where indicated.

Table 5.2 Salicylate content of various foods.*

Food	Salicylate content (mg per 100 g)	Typical portion	Salicylate intake (mg)
Fruits			
Cantaloupe melon	1.50	half (360 g)	4.68
Grapes	0.94	cluster (140 g)	1.32
Currants	5.80	2 handfuls (35 g)	2.03
Raisins	6.62	2 handfuls (30 g)	2.32
Grapefruit	0.68	6 segments (120 g)	0.82
Orange	2.39	1 (245 g)	5.86
Pineapple	2.10	1 slice (125 g)	2.63
Raspberries	5.14	15 (70 g)	3.60
Strawberry	1.6	1 serving (100 g)	1.60
Watermelon	0.48	1 slice (320 g)	2.46
Vegetables			
Broad beans	0.73	1 serving (75 g)	0.55
French beans	0.11	1 serving (105 g)	0.12
Broccoli	0.65	1 serving (95 g)	0.62
Parsnip	0.45	1 serving (110 g)	0.50
Spinach	0.58	1 serving (130 g)	0.75
Courgette/zucchini	1.04	1 serving (140 g)	1.46
Salads			
Chicory	1.02	1 serving (45 g)	0.46
Olive, green (canned)	1.29	9 (35 g)	0.45
Red pepper	1.20	1 serving (45 g)	0.54
Nuts			
Almonds	3.0	20 kernels (20 g)	0.60
Peanuts	1.12	32 (30 g)	0.34
Drinks			
Tea			
Breakfast	5.57	1 cup	5.57
Darjeeling	4.24	1 cup	4.24
Coffee			
Fresh beans	0.45	1 cup	0.45
Maxwell House	0.84	1 cup	0.84
Nescafé	0.59	1 cup	0.55

*For a fuller list, see Table A2.2, page 170.

have salicylate, but only in their skins, and the same is true of pears. Some unlikely foods can also be rich in salicylate, such as honey and products made from yeast, like savoury spreads and stock cubes. Drinks such as coffee and fruit juices contain salicylate, but the drink that has most is tea. Alcoholic drinks generally contain some salicylate, and this is the case with beer and wines, and especially with champagne and fortified wines such as port. Spirits like whisky and rum have a little, but there is none in gin or vodka.

The processing of certain foods can have a dramatic multiplier effect on salicylate. For example, while fresh tomatoes and tomato juice have 0.13 mg per 100 g, tomato soup has

0.54 mg, while tomato ketchup has 2.48 mg. Because salicylate is quite heat stable, process-ing will tend to concentrate the salicylate, which is why there is a lot in savoury spreads and gravy browning.

The information in Table 5.2 can be used to calculate the actual amount of salicylate a person would eat or drink at a given meal. This table has been worked out using typical size portions as given in the book *Nutrient Content of Food Portions*, by Jill Davies and John Dickerson. Together, Tables 5.1, 5.2, and A2.2 show how the menu at the start of this chapter could provide quite a lot of salicylate.

The salicylate in food is rapidly absorbed from the stomach and widely distributed round the body, and can be detected in joints, spinal fluid, and saliva. It can cross the pla-centa, but is lowest in brain and skeletal tissue. The body has mechanisms for removing this non-nutrient: some is broken down in the tissues, and these neutralised metabolic products are mainly excreted by the kidney into the urine. The majority of salicylate is excreted by the body unchanged.

Dr Ben Feingold was one of the first doctors to suggest that dietary salicylate could be sufficiently high to cause behavioural problems in children. He calculated that several hun-dred milligrams a day could be taken in from a diet rich in fruit and vegetables. In Australia, L. K. Salzman reported in the *Medical Journal of Australia* that the behaviour of hyperactive children improved following the removal of salicylate from their diet. This resulted in them becoming less easily distracted, less impulsive, and less excitable, and sleep and bed-wetting problems also improved. As very little salicylate crosses into the brain, the effect of reducing dietary salicylate is probably to reduce the levels of some more active compounds that are released by the pharmacological action of salicylate on cells. It is prob-ably these active compounds, rather than salicylate itself, which are responsible for these children's behaviour.

It is possible to avoid salicylate: Swain and her colleagues also discovered that several foods contain no salicylate at all. A salicylate-free diet need not lack variety, because it can include meat, vegetables, cereals, fruit, and dairy products (see Table 5.3).

Aspirin, rather than diet, is commonly the cause of salicylate intolerance problems in patients who have allergies such as asthma, rhinitis, and urticaria. They can be tested by measuring the levels of breakdown products after increasing doses of aspirin. Though the natural salicylates are rarely taken in levels high enough to produce this intolerance effect,

Table 5.3 Foods containing no salicylate.

Fruit	banana, pear (peeled)
Vegetables	lima beans, soya beans, green cabbage, celery lentils, potato (peeled), swede/yellow turnip, rice
Cereals	oats, wheat
Dairy products	cheddar cheese, cottage cheese, milk, cream yoghurt, eggs
Salads	lettuce
Meats and fish	beef, chicken, salmon, tuna
Others	soy sauce, cocoa, sugar, gin

it nevertheless can occur, and some patients, particularly those suffering from urticaria, do benefit from a diet low in natural salicylate.

Natural salicylates in medicine

Salicylate has been part of medical treatment for a long time. The Ebers papyrus, which dates from around 1500BC, is the oldest known medical reference work, and it lists 700 remedies that were in common use in ancient Egypt. One of them is a formula for treating inflammation, and it suggests crushed onion and honey in beer. As Table A2.2 in the Appendix shows, these three ingredients contain salicylate, and honey especially so. It might just have been possible for this remedy to provide enough salicylate to have an effect. But you would have needed to take nearly a kilogram of the most salicylate-rich honey just to give you the same amount of salicylate as you get in a junior aspirin tablet. Whatever the benefit this cure provided, it was not really ascribable to salicylate.

The papyrus also recommended an extract of willow bark as a way of treating those with infected wounds and high temperatures, and this was sensible advice: willow produces quite a lot of salicylate. A thousand years later this prescription was approved by Hippocrates (460–377BC), who was born on the Greek island of Cos and became the most highly regarded physician of the ancient world. He collected together all the medical science then known, and is reputed to have written 70 books. His advice was to drink an infusion of willow bark to alleviate the pain of childbirth. Both willow and poplar barks contain salicin, a salicylate derivative of glucose. While salicin is not aspirin, it has a close resemblance, both in its chemical structure and in its action in the body.

The great Roman physician and pharmacologist Dioscorides (AD40–90) wrote his influential work, *De materia medica*, in AD77. It is a list of over a thousand simple drugs and treatments, many of which had beneficial effects and were to be prescribed by doctors for over 1500 years. In his prescription for cooling a fever, Dioscorides advised coriander, a herb that contains salicylate. Again he was on the right lines, because salicylate is able to reduce body temperature; but as Table 5.1 shows, to gain any relief the patient would have to take a great deal of coriander.

In the seventeenth and eighteenth centuries, a theory called the doctrine of signatures became popular. This theory said that where a disease was prevalent, there nature would provide a cure. In the damp climate of the British Isles, rheumatism and rheumatic fever were common, and it was assumed that in the wettest regions there would be something to relieve these afflictions. One tree that thrives in a damp climate is the weeping willow, whose preferred habitat is marshy ground and the river bank. The Reverend Edmund Stone, an eighteenth-century English parson living in the Cotswolds, decided to investigate its bark. The bitterness of this pointed to the presence of an unusual substance. Stone, dried and powdered the willow bark, and gave an infusion of 20 grains (about 1 g) of it every four hours to people who had fever. He found they were much improved. He reported his findings to the Royal Society of London in 1763, and his letter is reproduced in the box. Stone had rediscovered Hippocrates' salicin, but had found a better use for it. Doctors started prescribing willow bark, while others wondered if the active ingredient itself could be extracted.

Rev Stone to the Royal Society   1763

My Lord,

There is a bark of an English tree which I have found by experience to be a powerful astringent and very efficacious in curing ague and intermitting disorders ... As this tree delights in a moist and wet soil where agues chiefly abound, the general maxim that many natural remedies carry their cures along with them ... was so very apposite in this case that I could not help applying it.

I determined to make some experiments with it and for the purpose I gathered near a pound weight of it, which I dried in a bag ... and reduced to a powder by pounding and sifting. I gave about twenty grains of powder at a dose and repeated it every four hours between fits ... The fits were considerably abated but did not entirely cease ... In a few days I increased the dose to two scruples and the ague was soon removed.

I then gave it to others with the same success, but I found it better answered the intention when a drachm of it was taken every four hours.

I have continued to use it as a remedy for ... five years successively and successfully. It hath been given to fifty persons and never failed in the cure except in a few autumnal and quartan agues with which the patient had been long and severely afflicted ...

To understand some of the terms in Stone's letter, you need to know that in those days the name for rheumatism was ague, and bouts of fever were called 'intermitting disorders'. The quantities he mentions are a grain, which is about 60 mg; a scruple, which is 20 grains and so around 1.2 g; and a drachm, which is 60 grains and about 4 g. We can not be certain how much salicin Stone's dried bark contained, but were it to be 10% by weight, then the drachm dose would be not much less than a modern adult-sized aspirin tablet.

In the 1820s an Italian chemist, Raffaele Piria, successfully isolated the chemical salicin, and from it he made salicylic acid itself. A few years later a Swiss chemist, Pagenstecher, discovered that salicin could also be extracted from the wild flower meadowsweet (*Spiraea ulmaria*). So why do plants make salicylate? In 1979 Raymond White at the Institute of Arable Crops Research at Rothamsted, Hertfordshire, England, discovered that injecting tobacco plants with salicylic acid prevented tobacco mosaic virus from attacking them. It was later shown that when a plant is infected, and even before the virus can be detected, the level of salicylate in the leaves rapidly increases five-fold. The salicylate is thought to act as a trigger to fire the plant into making a protein that it can use to fight the invader. Similar observations have been made with cucumbers, and it is probably a common defence mechanism in many plants. Oil of wintergreen, a popular embrocation and balm for aching

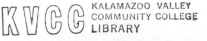

muscles, contains methyl salicylate. It is derived from the Pyrolaceae group of plants, and these are believed to produce methyl salicylate to counter insect attacks.

The aspirin story

A French chemist, Charles Frederic Gerhardt, had first made acetylsalicylic acid around 1850. It was tested as a painkiller and found to be very effective, but it had side-effects that ruled out its use: it burnt the mouth of those who tried it, and it tasted unpleasant. In 1893 the German chemist Felix Hoffmann was motivated by a desire to make a less unpleasant form of salicylic acid to treat his father's arthritis, and working with fellow chemist, Heinrich Dreser, he solved this problem. It transpired that the side-effects were caused by impurities, and so Hoffmann and Dreser found a way of purifying acetylsalicylic acid to yield a clean white powder which was not corrosive. It could be pressed into tablets, and these were easy to take and still had the potency of salicylic acid. Hoffmann and Dreser had made what would become one of the most successful proprietary drugs ever made, and one that was considered safe enough to be sold direct to the public. It was named Aspirin by their employer, the chemical company Bayer, but such was its popularity that this eventually became the generic name. It was called after the meadowsweet plant *Spiraea*, adding an 'a' for acetyl to get aspirin. Aspirin is still popular a century later: 25 000 tons are produced annually, and taken as 100 billion aspirin tablets every year around the world.

Aspirin is sold under scores of proprietary names, such as Anacin, Anadin, and Aspro. One version, Alka Seltzer, contains citric acid and sodium bicarbonate as well. The bicarbonate reacts with the aspirin to form its sodium salt, thereby making it soluble in water and supposedly quicker acting and gentler on the stomach. The bicarbonate also reacts with some of the citric acid to generate bubbles of carbon dioxide, and the citric acid gives the final drink a pleasant fruit-like flavour.

All the soluble forms of aspirin are the sodium or calcium salts of acetylsalicylic acid, which dissolve readily in water to give a clear liquid which some people prefer to drink and easier to take than a tablet. However, once it reaches the stomach the acid conditions there immediately turn these chemicals back to the insoluble form, although this is now as very fine crystals which are less irritating to the lining of the stomach than particles of a large tablet.

Other forms of aspirin are combined with caffeine, which has a synergistic effect (in other words each reinforces the effect of the other), or with aluminium hydroxide and magnesium hydroxide, which are antacids and may prevent the stomach irritation, or in slow release formulations. But whatever form of aspirin you take, in the body it always becomes salicylic acid.

An aspirin a day keeps the doctor away

Aspirin deadens pain, lessens inflammation, reduces fevers, and prevents the blood from clotting. It does all this by controlling a group of body chemicals known as prostaglandins, which are produced in response to injury. To be on the safe side, our body generally makes too much prostaglandin, and the result is experienced as aches, pains, high temperatures, and soreness. Because of its influence on this wide range of symptoms, aspirin has gained a popular reputation for being good for almost every common ailment, be it asthma or arthritis, flu or fibrositis, sore throat or sore arm, headache or hangover, pulled muscle or period pain—take a couple of aspirins and you will soon feel better.

There are other claims for the benefits of aspirin; for example, in cases of senile dementia it keeps up the flow of blood to the brain. It may be able to destroy free radicals, those super-active natural chemicals that are formed within the body and which are thought to initiate cancer (see the Glossary). A report in the US *Annals of Internal Medicine* in 1994 showed that in a group of 48 000 men, tracked over a period of eight years, those who had been using aspirin for a number of years were far less likely to contract colon and rectal cancer. Aspirin also prevents cataracts because it counters the proteins that make the lens of the eye opaque. It has also been shown to reduce the severity of withdrawal symptoms, mainly convulsions, in alcoholic mice, and it may do the same in humans.

In the 1950s there was anecdotal evidence that that aspirin might protect people against heart attacks. This suggestion, which was dismissed at the time, was eventually to become part of the accepted treatment for heart patients. It has long been a puzzling fact that while the French have a diet rich in animal fats, they also have one of the lowest rates of heart disease in the world. The French paradox seemed to contradict the perceived wisdom that animal fats, which contain a lot of saturated fat, were harmful to the heart and cause ill health. The recommended dietary advice in many countries was to avoid animal fats such as butter, cream, and lard, and to replace them with vegetable oils and especially monounsaturated oils, such as olive oil. But French people's hearts seemed none the worse for their diet, and it became an accepted truth that they somehow were taking in something else that was protecting them.

In his research into heart disease and its links with diet, Professor S. Renaud, Director of INSERM, Bion, France, studied the people of two cities with similar populations: Toulouse, the regional centre in the south of France, and Belfast in Northern Ireland. The residents of Belfast were dying of heart disease at four times the rate of those in Toulouse. Wine, and especially red wine, was suggested as an explanation. This theory was put forward in the USA in 1992 by a group at the Kaiser Medical Center in Oakland, California, giving a healthy fillip to wine sales across North America.

But Rernaud thought there might be another reason, and that was that the residents of Toulouse ate far more fresh fruit and vegetables than the people in Belfast. They were getting a diet much richer in salicylate.

In 1994 the *British Medical Journal* announced the results of 300 clinical trials around the world on 140 000 patients who had experienced a heart attack, angina, a stroke, or surgery for blocked coronary arteries. The results were analysed by a team of international scientists from 28 countries, including Australia, Argentina, Brazil, Canada, China, France, Germany, India, Italy, Japan, Thailand, the UK, and the USA, and they showed that taking aspirin regularly can cut heart attacks by a quarter in high-risk patients. They were also able to say that aspirin worked irrespective of sex, age, blood pressure, or blood sugar (glucose) levels. This evidence contradicted previous suggestions that women, old people, those with high blood pressure and diabetics may not benefit from taking aspirin.

Aspirin interferes with enzymes that make precursors to the prostaglandins—the hormones that control processes such as inflammation, digestion, kidney function, reproduction, and blood clotting. It is this last effect that explains how aspirin may reduce the likelihood of strokes and heart attacks. The prostaglandins cause blood platelets to aggregate together, forming a blood clot. Platelets start the repair of damaged blood vessels, and this they do by forming an immediate film over the hole, on top of which a blood clot forms, plugging the wound. Part of a clot may be dislodged and move to block vital arteries, causing a stroke, if the blockage is in the brain, or a heart attack if it is in the heart. Aspirin reduces levels of prostaglandins in the body, making it less likely that these dangerous clots will form.

The prostaglandins also alert the body to damage, and this often leads to uncomfortable symptoms such as inflammation, fever and pain when the amount produced is excessive.

A sequence of chemical reactions leads to the appearance of prostaglandins, and the first is the liberation of arachidonic acid from a damaged cell membrane. In the presence of an enzyme this acid reacts with oxygen to form prostaglandin precursors, and these trigger inflammation. Aspirin blocks the enzyme, and so controls the chain of events that starts with a damaged cell and leads eventually to soreness or pain, thus reducing our discomfort while our body heals.

Body temperature is regulated in the part of the brain known as the hypothalamus, and this too is controlled by prostaglandins. This is why aspirin is good at reducing high temperatures. While a high temperature may be part of the body's defence against a bacterial and viral attack, it can lead to organ damage if it goes too high.

Although aspirin has been used for many years, it is not without its risks. Were it to be discovered today, it would never be approved for common use because it causes stomach bleeding in a significant percentage of people. For this reason you would be well advised to consult your doctor before taking it regularly. Aspirin also presents a more serious risk: for some young children it can be fatal if they are given it to treat the viral infections of influenza and chicken pox. They can develop Reye's syndrome, the symptoms of which include confusion, irrational behaviour, delirium, convulsions, and coma. The condition is fatal in about half the cases, if liver and brain damage is severe, although early treatment can cut the death rate to around 10%. For this reason children under the age of 12 should never be prescribed aspirin. Reye's syndrome is, however, a very rare condition.

Despite its disadvantages, aspirin is still a remarkable drug, and much more than just a painkiller. It protects against heart disease, thrombosis, cataracts, and senile dementia, and has even been mooted as a possible treatment for cancer. If you suffer no stomach pain with aspirin and you are in a high risk category for heart disease, then you might be well be advised by your doctor to take a small aspirin tablet every day.

But what should you do if you think you are sensitive to salicylate? If taking an aspirin causes stomach pain, then you might be one of the unlucky few who should avoid foods with high levels of salicylate. In which case, you might well find the following menu more to your taste.

Salicylate-free MENU

Starter	Smoked salmon
Main courses	Chicken Kiev
	Beef Stroganoff
	Macaroni cheese
	All served with French fries or rice
Dessert	Banana split with chocolate sauce and ice cream

CHAPTER 6

Caffeine

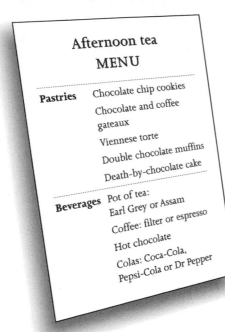

Afternoon tea
MENU

Pastries   Chocolate chip cookies
Chocolate and coffee
gateaux
Viennese torte
Double chocolate muffins
Death-by-chocolate cake

Beverages Pot of tea:
Earl Grey or Assam
Coffee: filter or espresso
Hot chocolate
Colas: Coca-Cola,
Pepsi-Cola or Dr Pepper

Treat yourself from the above menu and you could take in enough caffeine to give yourself a real caffeine 'buzz.' And why not? You would only be doing what humans have done for thousands of years.

The earliest written record of human use of caffeine is from China around 2700 BC, which is about tea-drinking. Coffee came much later: it was cultivated first in the sixth century AD in Ethiopia, and then in Turkey, where it acquired the name kahveh, from which the words coffee, café, and, ultimately, caffeine, were to be derived. Meanwhile in North America, caffeine-containing beverages were being made from guarana, yoco, and maté in the south, and from cassina in the north; while in Central and South America cocoa was drunk, which also contains caffeine. In Africa, the popular way to partake of caffeine was to chew kola nuts.

Caffeine is produced by many different kinds of trees, bushes, flowers, and even cacti. More than a hundred plants generate this molecule, though why they do so is still a mystery. One theory is that caffeine protects the plants from attack by insects; perhaps it does, but the evidence is not compelling—both tea and coffee growers still need to use commercial insecticides to protect their crops from insect pests. However, of all these plants, only three produce caffeine in amounts that make harvesting them a commercial possibility: tea, coffee, and cocoa. The caffeine content of coffee beans is 0.8–1.8% by weight; for fresh leaves from the tea plant it is 0.7–2.1%; and for cocoa beans it is 1–2%.

These crops were developed because of the beneficial effects that they produced when they were drunk as infusions, and today we consume caffeine on a vast scale: half the world's population regularly drinks tea, a third drinks coffee, and a large proportion drinks colas.

Worldwide consumption of caffeine is now estimated to be over 120 000 tons per year, which works out at about 60 mg per person per day. Scandinavians have the largest caffeine intake, generally from coffee, with over 400 mg per day; the British consume around 300 mg per day, much of it as tea; and the Americans, long regarded as big coffee and cola drinkers, get a surprisingly low 200 mg per day. Most young people get their daily dose of caffeine from colas, whereas most adults get it from coffee and tea. Tea is mainly drunk in the countries in which it is grown, such as India, Sri Lanka, and especially China. On the other hand, coffee is mainly grown as a crop for export in countries like Brazil, Colombia, Indonesia, and Kenya. International trade in coffee beans exceeds $7 billion a year, making them one of the world's major bulk-traded commodities.

Caffeine is present as a drug in hundreds of products, such as painkillers, pick-me-ups, and dietary aids, as well as in medicinal treatments like diuretics and asthma relief preparations. It has a synergistic effect with some painkillers, such as paracetamol (also known as acetaminophen, and sold as Tylenol in the USA). This means that the amount of the painkilling drug can be reduced by 40% and yet still provide the same degree of relief when it is boosted by caffeine. The popular painkiller Anacin (also known as Anadin) contains 32 mg of caffeine per tablet.

Caffeine is a non-nutrient, and it affects different people in different ways. Some people even experience withdrawal symptoms when they go without caffeine-containing drinks for more than a couple of days. But is it safe? In 1980 the US Food and Drug Administration felt it had to advise pregnant women to reduce their intake of caffiene, when it was proved that when they had a caffeine-containing drink, they passed some of the drug to the unborn baby. Caffeine can cross the placenta, and it has been shown to cause birth defects in test animals, although at doses far higher than any human would experience.

But most people need not worry that consuming caffeine is dangerous. The recommended maximum daily intake is 250 mg, but there is no scientific evidence that even 300 mg a day of this natural chemical can do us any harm, and that is equivalent to four cups of strong coffee, or six cans of cola, or eight cups of tea, or a dozen bars of chocolate. Indeed, many of the innocent rituals for coping with stress involve caffeine, such as relaxing over a cup of tea or coffee, refreshing oneself with a can of cola, or rewarding oneself with a piece of chocolate confectionery.

So how much caffeine do we get when we drink coffee, tea, or cola? The amounts are very variable. In coffee it depends on the species of bean: *Coffea robusta* is the variety grown in West Africa and Indonesia, and it contains slightly more caffeine than *Coffea arabica*, which is grown in East Africa, the Caribbean, and Central and South America.

The amount of caffeine also depends on whether we are using instant or ground coffee, and if the latter, on how we make it—by percolator or filter. There is more caffeine in strong

Table 6.1 The amount of caffeine in various kinds of drink.

Source	Caffeine content of typical size (mg) portions*	Average content (mg)
Instant coffee	40–100	60
Ground coffee	60–120	80
Decaffeinated coffee	2–8	5
Tea	30–55	40
Cola	35–60	40
Hot chocolate (cocoa)	2–7	5/10**
Chocolate bar	20	20/40**

*When drinking coffee, tea, and hot chocolate people either use a cup of 150 mls (6 ounces) or a mug of around 200 mls (8 ounces), which is why there is a range of values for these drinks. For cola the standard is a can of 330 mls (12 ounces), and for chocolate it is a bar of 100 grams (3.5 ounces).
**Chocolate also contains theobromine and this is also like caffeine in its effects and is roughly equivalent to doubling the amount of caffeine, to 10 mg in cup of hot chocolate, and 40 mg in chocolate candy.

coffee than in weak coffee. In tea, the amount of caffeine also depends on the strength of the drink, but in colas it depends on the brand we drink. Table 6.1 gives the average intake when we take a shot of caffeine.

Coffee

The wonderful aroma of fresh coffee comes from a mix of some 2000 different chemicals, many of which are still to be identified. But it is not the aroma or taste of coffee that accounts for its popularity: it is the caffeine it contains.

A cup of instant coffee provides 60 mg of caffeine, and over the past 50 years, this has become the most popular way to drink it. The Brazilian Institute for Coffee showed in 1930 that coffee could be reduced to a soluble powder, and instant coffee was first produced by the Swiss company, Nestlé, in 1938 and sold as Nescafé. Instant coffee really came into its own in World War II when it was widely used by US troops. Thereafter it became part of everyday living.

There are many popular misconceptions about coffee. It is accused of causing sleepless nights, indigestion, and bad breath, as well as heart disease. In fact it does not cause insomnia, indigestion, or heart disease in the majority of drinkers, and this was the conclusion of 175 scientists from around the world who attended the International Caffeine Workshop in Greece in 1993. Nevertheless, it does affect some people, as the box explains.

Case histories: **Coffee dreams**

There can be a ten-fold difference between individuals in the rate at which caffeine is detoxified and eliminated from their bodies. Thus one person will be quickly rid of his or her stimulating after-dinner coffee and be asleep before midnight, whereas the slow metaboliser is still awake in the early hours. Those who are affected this way soon learn to limit their caffeine intake to early in the day.

In Stephen Braun's delightful book *Buzz*, which is about alcohol and caffeine, he tells the strange stories of three people for whom coffee had exactly the opposite effect to the one most people experience. No matter how much they drank, they kept falling asleep.

A 35-year-old office worker drank 10 cups of coffee and two litres of cola a day, equivalent to more than 800 mg of caffeine, yet she still slept 12 hours each night and often fell asleep in front of the television in the evening. A 52-year-old secretary drank coffee many times a day, and still found it hard to keep awake in the afternoon. A 45-year-old man drank seven cups of coffee a day, and took caffeine pills because he was always sleepy: he even fell asleep at meal times.

All were advised to give up caffeine, and in all three cases their symptoms disappeared. For them caffeine was a depressant, not the stimulant it is for most people.

Decaffeinated coffee ('decaff') was first produced by the German company Kaffee HAG in the early 1900s, but it was only after a series of scares in the 1970s and 1980s, linking the caffeine of coffee to various diseases, that demand for it grew. People turned to decaff because they feared that caffeine was a health risk, although, as we shall see, drinking decaff in those days was probably more risky. When the charge against caffeine proved to be unfounded, decaffeinated coffee sales in the USA began to decline, from a high of 17% of all coffee purchases at the height of the coffee scares in the early 1980s, to around 12% today. Even so, this is still much higher than sales before the coffee scares began, when fewer than 5% drank decaff. Such is still the demand for decaff in the USA that it adds $1 billion annually to the cost of processing coffee. For this reason there is a great deal of interest in the researches at the US biotechnology company Integrated Coffee Technologies, where the first genetically modified plant that produces a caffeine-free coffee bean was announced in 1997. The main beneficiaries of this would be those who love the flavour of coffee, but who find it hard to deal with the caffeine it contains.

John Stiles and colleagues at the University of Hawaii, in Manoa, have developed the new beans. They first identified the master gene that codes for caffeine production, and then blocked its function with an anti-sense gene. The plants which grew from tissue cultures showed only 3% of the normal amount of caffeine.

Tea

The Emperor Shen Nung in 2737BC was the first person of note to recognise the benefits of drinking tea. This habit has continued for thousands of years, in the belief that tea not only cheered you up, but was also good for your health. There may be some truth in this, as we shall see.

'Wouldn't it be dreadful to live in a country where they didn't have tea?' wrote Noel Coward. He was of course referring to the custom that came to represent an essential part of the British way of life: the ritual of afternoon tea. Not surprisingly, tea is still widely drunk in former parts of the Empire, and especially the UK, Australia, New Zealand, Canada, and Ireland, as well as in those former colonies in which it is grown: India, Kenya, Pakistan, and Ceylon. Tea was also decidedly rejected by those who broke away from the Empire, such as the American colonists, where in 1773 a group of protesters deliberately destroyed a cargo of tea in what became known as the Boston Tea Party. Abstaining from tea came to symbolise defiance against the despised British, and coffee took its place.

Tea comes in two basic forms, green and black, and both are from the leaves of the plant *Camellia sinensis*. Green tea is made by steaming the leaves the day they are harvested, and this keeps them green. Black tea is made by allowing the leaves to wither, after which they are rolled and crushed to start the oxidation processes. There is a second kind of black tea, the oolong tea that is drunk in southern China, in which the oxidation is prevented by heating the leaves immediately after rolling.

All teas contain caffeine, plus lots of other molecules called polyphenols, of which the most abundant are the flavanols (known as catechins in the trade). In black tea the flavanols have been oxidised to theaflavins and thearubigins. Black tea also contains unoxidised polyphenols, which have antioxidant properties that are thought to protect cells against damage caused by free radicals (see the Glossary). While all teas are excellent sources of unoxidised polyphenols green tea has five times as much as black tea.

One polyphenol in particular, called epigallocathechin-3 gallate (or EGCG for short), inhibits the enzyme urokinase, which plays an important role in the growth of malignant cells. EGCG's beneficial effects, and those of green tea, were reported by Jerzy Jankun and colleagues, of the University of Toledo, Ohio, USA, in the journal *Nature* in 1997. The flavanols in tea will prevent *N*-nitroso compounds from forming in the body, and these are potent cancer-forming chemicals. Janelle Landau and Chung Yang, of Rutgers University, New Jersey, USA, report that cancer in special mice, which are bred to be highly susceptible to lung cancer, is inhibited by tea, and by green tea especially. Tests on these mice have also shown that tea reduces the risk of stomach, intestine, and colon cancers, and that green tea is particularly beneficial.

Not surprisingly, green tea extracts are now being added to all kinds of products, such as cleansing lotions, skin moisturisers, chewing gum, and even toothpaste, despite the lack of hard evidence that they will confer any benefits on those who buy them. Substances that can be demonstrated to have an effect *in vitro*, in other words in laboratory experiments, may not necessarily have the same effect *in vivo*, in other words in living things. Indeed, they rarely do. But outside the laboratory, epidemiological studies also indicate the benefits of tea drinking. The antioxidants in tea may explain the findings of Michael Hertog in the Netherlands, who discovered that the risk of heart attacks and stroke went down, the more tea people drank. A Japanese survey has shown that people who drink green tea have lower cholesterol levels than those who do not. However, a similar study in Wales found no such relationship between black tea and health, prompting the suggestions that adding milk to tea, which is how it is drunk in Wales, robbed the tea of its antioxidant properties.

While some epidemiological surveys reveal the benefits of tea-drinking among humans, other surveys have uncovered no positive benefits at all. For example, one survey found that tea conferred benefit against bladder cancer, but 18 other surveys could not confirm this. In the case of stomach cancer, two reports documented less stomach cancer among tea-drinkers, while five others actually found such people to be *more* likely to develop the disease, and 14 further surveys could not confirm a strong link either way.

Whether tea inhibits the formation and growth of cancers is still being debated. Nevertheless, the lower rates of cancer, and other diseases, in China have been attributed to the benefits of drinking green tea, six cups a day of which would provide a dose of 900 mg of EGCG. However, it is not the polyphenols that we seek when we drink a cup of tea, but the caffeine. Chemically these compounds are not related, nor do they interfere with one another, and if some components of tea offer us health benefits as well, then that is a bonus.

Colas

The most popular drink in the USA is carbonated water in the form of fruit-flavoured sodas and colas. The average person drinks 3.5 litres (roughly a US gallon) a week, compared to 2.5 litres of coffee. Of the carbonated drinks, 86% contain caffeine, and of these Coca-Cola, Pepsi-Cola, and Dr Pepper make up the majority. These were concocted in the USA in the 1880s, and have become universal best-sellers.

Most ingredients in colas have been criticised at one time or another. Examine the label on a bottle or can, and it appears that all you are drinking is a solution of chemicals in fizzy water. Little that they contain can be described as wholesome: the main ingredients are sugar (or an artificial sweetener), phosphoric acid, caffeine, and a blend of supposedly secret flavourings. Despite this—indeed, because of it—Coca-Cola has been highly successful and billions of cans are sold every week around the world.

The story of Coca-Cola began in June 1887 in Atlanta, Georgia, when a pharmacist, Dr John Pemberton, placed an advertisement in the *Atlanta Journal* describing a new drink he had concocted:

> *Delicious! Refreshing! Exhilarating! Invigorating!*
> *The new and popular soda fountain drink contains the properties of*
> *the wonderful coca plant and the famous cola nut.*

The drink was named Coca-Cola after these ingredients. The coca plant provided a little cocaine, and the cola nut some caffeine. Neither of these plants provides ingredients for today's cola, and the cocaine component was removed soon after the drink was launched. The time was right for the new beverage, because the city of Atlanta had just voted to ban alcohol within the city limits. But Pemberton's new drink continued to sell well even after that local prohibition law was repealed later that year.

Pemberton had devised a recipe that was to become the world's best-selling soft drink. He kept its ingredients a closely guarded secret at the time, but the main ones were sugar, caramel, caffeine, phosphoric acid, lime juice, and vanilla essence. The acidity of Coca-Cola, which was needed for its refreshing taste, was originally due to citric acid, which occurs in citrus fruits, but this ingredient was soon replaced with cheaper phosphoric acid. Pemberton needed to make his new drink distinctive, so he experimented with other flavours, but in smaller amounts. For over a hundred years Coca-Cola refused to divulge his recipe, but it was discovered by chance in one of Pemberton's note books: we now know that his secret concoction was a blend of the oils of lemon, orange, nutmeg, cinnamon, neroli, and coriander.

There are people who say that they can identify the different colas that are available, and it appears that when they are offered a choice in a blind-fold test they usually say they prefer Pepsi-Cola, although Coca-Cola outsells its main rival by a large margin. Even so, they are both relatively expensive if you want a shot of caffeine. The amount of caffeine in a can of cola or soft drink varies according to brand:

Mountain Dew	57 mg
Coca-Cola	48 mg
Diet Coke	48 mg
Dr Pepper	42 mg
Pepsi-Cola	41 mg
Diet Pepsi	38 mg

In some countries there is a limit to the amount of caffeine allowed in a can of cola: in Australia, the maximum is 55 mg per 375 ml can. As the above figures show, it is not difficult to exceed the recommended maximum intake of caffeine of 250 mg per day if you drink lots of cola.

Chocolate

Chocolate comes from the beans of the cacao tree. While the beans contain a lot less caffeine than coffee beans, they make up for this by having a lot more of another caffeine-like chemical called theophylline—up to seven times as much. This means there is around 500 mg of theophylline in a 100 g bar of chocolate. Although theophylline is less potent, it still has the same overall effect as caffeine. Like tea, chocolate contains other chemicals that can affect us, including phenylethylamine, the biogenic amine that was discussed in Chapter 5. This amine may account for the cravings of those who say they are chocoholics. These people are generally women, who find that chocolate is irresistible, especially before their monthly period. Although chocolate contains many active chemicals, some of which may mimic natural hormones, none of these is addictive.

The popular varieties of chocolate consist of 8% protein, 60% carbohydrate, and 30% fat, although this last component is at the upper limit of what is desirable. A normal 100 g (3½ ounce) bar provides 520 calories, but it also provides some essential minerals, especially potassium, calcium, iron, copper, and zinc, and vitamins A, B_1, B_2, niacin, and E. Looking at this list of ingredients, it is perhaps not surprising that chocolate bars make excellent emergency rations for soldiers and explorers, providing mainly energy; but there are a few things missing, like vitamins C and D, so it is far from being a complete food.

The Mayas, who flourished in Mexico from AD250 to 900, discovered the benefits of chocolate, which they took as a drink, but it was reserved for the ruling elite. By the time the Spaniards arrived in Mexico at the end of the fifteenth century, the Aztec Empire was at its height, and its economy was partly based on cocoa beans, Aztec nobles reserved chocolate drinking for themselves, regarding it as an aphrodisiac. When cocoa beans were taken back to Europe, they went with the reputation of a love-stimulant, and this remained a popular belief into the eighteenth century, when the great lover, Casanova, proclaimed chocolate to be his preferred drink.

Cocoa beans are harvested from the cacao tree, Theobroma cacoa ('theobroma' means 'food of the gods'). These trees grow best in warm, moist climates and within 20 degrees of latitude from the Equator. They are grown in Brazil and Mexico, for the North American market, and in West Africa for the European market. World production of cocoa beans is two million tons a year.

After cocoa pods are harvested, the beans are left in the sun to ferment. This exposure turns them brown and converts some of their sugars first into alcohol and then to acetic acid, which we know best in the form of vinegar. Phenylethylamine also forms during this fermentation stage. The beans are then roasted which generates the flavour compounds and removes most of the acetic acid. They are then milled, which melts the cocoa fat.

Today when we speak of chocolate, we think of a chocolate bar, but for over 250 years in Europe, chocolate was taken as a drink. The name is derived from the Aztec word xocolatl, meaning bitter water, and people drank it mixed with cinnamon and cornmeal. Europeans used vanilla and sugar to make it sweeter and more palatable. The transformation of chocolate from a drink to a confectionery bar began in 1847, when the Quaker confectioners, J. S. Fry & Sons, of Bristol, England, introduced a solid form that could be eaten as a sweet. They made it by pressing molten chocolate to squeeze out the cocoa butter, and then added this to more molten chocolate. When it cooled down the mixture set to give what we now call plain chocolate or cooking chocolate, which has rather a strong flavour. Milk chocolate was first produced in 1876 by the chemist Henri Nestlé: he added condensed milk, which made the product lighter in taste and colour. Other Quaker families, such as the Cadburys, the Rowntrees, and the Hersheys, entered the chocolate business, and went on to establish large chocolate empires in the UK and the USA.

Despite what people have thought, chocolate is not an aphrodisiac; but three of its components certainly affect the brain: theobromine and caffeine act in the same way, and in a manner explained below, while phenylethylamine probably raises the level of glucose in the blood and triggers the release of dopamine, as described in a previous chapter.

Of the common sources of caffeine, chocolate has the least, and if you are one of those people susceptible to this non-nutrient then you would be better advised to give up drinking coffee, colas, and tea rather than deny yourself the occasional enjoyment of chocolate.

What is caffeine and how does it work?

Pure caffeine is a white powder. It was first isolated in 1820 by a German chemist called Friedlieb Runge, and its molecular structure was deduced in 1897. It can be made in the laboratory, but the commercial market is more than amply supplied by the caffeine that is produced as a by-product of decaffeinating coffee.

Caffeine is known chemically as 1,3,7-trimethyl-xanthine. This means that it has xanthine as its core molecule, and attached to that are three methyl groups (CH_3), on atoms 1, 3, and 7. There are also very similar molecules with only two methyls, and these can be on atoms 1 and 3, or 1 and 7, or 3 and 7. These molecules tend also to be present naturally where there is caffeine. They are called theophylline, paraxanthine, and theobromine respectively, and behave similarly to caffeine, except that theophylline is slightly more powerful than caffeine while theobromine is less powerful.

What effect does caffeine have on our body? Popular impressions are that caffeine keeps us awake and sobers us up. Research shows that its effects are much more subtle.

Caffeine is metabolised by the liver, which takes about 12 hours to remove 90% of any caffeine we have consumed. How it affects us depends on our body weight, and also on how long it has been since we last had a caffeine-based drink. The first few times that we have caffeine, it puts up our heart rate and blood pressure quite dramatically, but as we become regular drinkers of colas, coffee, and tea, our body no longer reacts in this way. Yet caffeine is a stimulant, and its drinks used to be advertised to emphasise this, so we were told that coffee wakes us up, colas refresh, and a cup of tea revives.

Caffeine does have other effects. People given doses of 250 and 500 mg of caffeine were observed to have shaky hands—a symptom that peaked after about an hour and lasted for about two hours. The effect varied very much from individual to individual, and it is this variability that has puzzled many researchers into the effects of caffeine. Many people take in caffeine daily, sometimes in quite high doses, so tolerance to it must be quite high. Consequently a dose of 250 mg will be far in excess of some people's regular intake, but well within the level that others are accustomed to. In experiments to test whether caffeine could produce anxiety neurosis it was necessary to give doses of over 1000 mg per day on a regular basis. The result was that at this level caffeine did indeed lead to symptoms often associated with anxiety, such as nervousness, insomnia, sensory disturbances, irritability, and trembling.

Athletes use caffeine to boost their performance, but it can exact a high price, as Sylvia Gerasch discovered. She was the European 100-metre breast-stroke champion, but in January 1994 she tested positive for caffeine and was duly stripped of her title and banned from competitive events for two years. She had 16 mg per litre of caffeine in her blood, which was well over the limit of 12 mg set by the authorities. This level could be achieved by drinking lots of strong coffee in the half-hour before an event. To have reached 16 mg, Gerasch would have had to have taken in around 750 mg of the drug (or drunk six cups of strong coffee) before the race.

Research at Christ Church College, Canterbury, England, showed that runners who took 350 mg of caffeine before a 1500-metre race improved their time by around four seconds on average—which may not sound much, but may be enough to win. Those taking part in cycle races drink caffeine both before and during the race, and some even insert caffeine supposi-tories to release the drug slowly. Caffeine promotes the conversion of stored body fat into energy, so that this reserve becomes available in addition to the energy stored as carbohydrate. It has been suggested that caffeine affects the enzymes that control the glycogen (energy) store, but how it achieves this is not yet fully understood. The extra energy is certainly a use-ful boost during endurance-type sporting events. Caffeine also appears to promote the release of calcium into brain tissue and muscles. These theories help explain the popular idea that caffeine makes you more active and alert.

Caffeine is not only a pick-me-up: it also has medicinal benefits, and is used in painkillers, asthma treatments, and diet aids, although this last use is now banned in certain countries such as the USA where it was outlawed in 1991 by the Food and Drug Administration. Caffeine aids dieting partly because it is a mild diuretic and laxative, and partly because it boosts the body's metabolism, encouraging it to burn more fat when we exercise. Caffeine acts in these ways by interfering with adenosine. It stimulates urination by blocking the adenosine receptors in the kidneys, where there are lots of them. This makes the blood vessels there dilate, which means that the kidneys can filter more blood. It stimulates the colon, which also has lots of adenosine receptors that tend to restrain the functioning of the muscles of the gut wall.

Adenosine sedates, kills pain, and calms brain activity. It is present in all tissues, and damps down neurotransmitters, which is why we feel tired when adenosine is released in the brain. As neurons trigger, adenosine is produced and occupies receptors that are embedded into the neuron membranes (and other tissues). This slows down the neuron's firing rate. While we rest or sleep the adenosine levels fall, allowing neuron activity to build up again.

Adenosine also regulates functions such as blood pressure and heart beat as well as brain activity. This is why caffeine affects blood pressure, and can boost cardiac output by as much as 50%—but only if we take in 10 mg per kilogram of body weight, which is around 700 mg for the average person. (Cardiac output is the product of stroke volume and pulse rate; caffeine increases both.) This would be like drinking 12 cups of strong coffee one after the other. At this sort of level caffeine increases the heart rate, raises the blood pressure, increases anxiety, and reduces the blood flow to the brain. However, the effects depend very much on the person, and on their previous use of caffeine-types drinks; and in some cases the effect can be delayed for over an hour. Caffeine also makes muscles contract more eas-ily, and it makes breathing easier. Caffeine's close relative theophylline is prescribed for bronchial asthma in adult doses of 250 mg, which is enough to relax the bronchial passage-ways and ease breathing.

Caffeine molecules can fit into the adenosine receptors, but it is the wrong shape to trig-ger them, so it prevents the receptor passing back the message to slow down. Everywhere in the body that adenosine has a calming role, caffeine can counter it. So far three different types of adenosine receptor have been identified, but it is not yet certain that caffeine can block all of them. However, it is possible that adenosine receptors are the solution to the puzzle of why different people react differently to the same dose of caffeine: they may have different numbers and distributions of adenosine receptors.

Work by Lydia Conlay and colleagues of MIT, Cambridge, Massachusetts, published in *Nature* in 1997, showed that caffeine increases the adenosine in the blood plasma of rats in direct proportion to the amount of caffeine up to a certain level. Once that level was reached, there was no further increase, despite an increase in the amount of caffeine taken. The rats were allowed unlimited access to a 0.1% solution of caffeine, and were observed to take in about 40 mg per day, which would be equivalent to a human taking in around 4500 mg a day. Adenosine levels shot up from 0.3 μM to 3 μM (μM is a measure of concentration), but once caffeine was withdrawn it fell to 0.1 μM, which is below their normal level. The authors of this paper calculated that caffeine, at the levels at which most coffee-drinkers take it in (around 500 mg per day if they drink 6 cups), would also experience a change in adenosine levels. Heavy coffee drinkers may have 12 cups a day, and they would get 1000 mg of caffeine. Were they suddenly to stop drinking coffee at this level, then their adenosine level would also plummet, and this could trigger bronchospasm, alter blood pressure, change heart rhythms, and influence seizure thresholds.

Caffeine is not acting as a stimulator itself, but it obstructs the action of adenosine which would slow activity down. Clearly the most that caffeine can do is to block all adenosine receptors and ensure that the body's neurotransmitters are working to their full capacity. For this reason it is difficult to overdose on caffeine, although there is a case of death from an accidental caffeine injection, when 3200 mg was given. The fatal overdose by mouth is probably around 5000 mg.

Caffeine molecules will generally occupy up to half the adenosine receptors, and thereby interfere with adenosine's ability to regulate some key functions, which is why caffeine has some of the effects claimed for it. And it does not take much to produce these effects: as little as one cup of coffee will suffice—indeed, higher doses have relatively less effect. Consequently it is not surprising that those who wish to carry out clinical investigations on the drug caffeine may find it almost impossible to do so, because even the small intakes of the drug, unbeknown to the doctor and overlooked by the patient, may interfere with the tests.

In the 1970s there was much concern that caffeine was responsible for coronary heart disease. An epidemiological survey seemed to bear this out, and the Boston Collaborative Surveillance Program of 1972 announced that those people who drank more than six cups of coffee a day were twice as likely to suffer a heart attack as people in general. This was supported by a further survey which covered more than 12 000 individuals and took into account variations arising from gender, age, blood pressure, obesity, smoking, and other suspected risk factors. However, these epidemiological surveys were not supported by later analysis, and other studies over the next 15 years failed to confirm this supposed link between heart disease and coffee drinking. For example, a large survey was carried out in Scotland, where there is a particularly high incidence of heart disease in both men and women. The researchers questioned more than 10 000 middle-aged men and women and could find no link between caffeine intake and heart disease.

Epidemiological surveys may sometimes be compromised by the quality of the data that are gathered, and the way they are analysed. Great care must be taken to ensure that unseen factors do not unduly influence their findings, and this is not easy to achieve when there is little control over the group that is being investigated. Those unskilled in the methodology of carrying out epidemiological surveys may introduce unsuspected bias into the way they collect the data, or be unaware of significant details which have an influence on those data. This appears to have been the case in some of the early surveys into coffee drinking and possible links to disease. In several cases the original findings, showing such links, could not be corroborated by those who later carried out much more detailed surveys. Unfortunately, the publicity given to the original findings caused public alarm, and led to unnecessary worry and changes in drinking habits that offered no real benefit. For example, one of the most serious of the surveys was published in the early 1980s in the prestigious *New England Journal of Medicine*. The report claimed that there was a statistical link between drinking more than five cups of coffee a day and developing cancer of the pancreas. This is a disease for which there is no treatment, and which is rapidly fatal. The news made headlines around the world, and the bottom fell out of the coffee market. Subsequent studies failed to support the original paper, and it was later suggested that the original workers had overlooked a confounding variable, in this case decaffeinated coffee. Residual traces of the solvent used to decaffeinate coffee were found in the product, and the solvent then in use was known to produce cancers in laboratory mice.

Because it has known physiological effects, it is not surprising that caffeine has been thought to be a factor in some common diseases. A survey in 1973 suggested that the risk of thrombosis was doubled if a person consumed 400 mg a day, equivalent to drinking five cups of fresh coffee. However, a study in 1990 on 45 000 men failed to find any connection between thrombosis and coffee drinking. As more and more data have been collected and analysed, the many scares about caffeine have been shown to be little more than the artefacts of poorly designed epidemiological studies into people's eating habits.

Getting rid of caffeine

Caffeine circulates in the bloodstream and diffuses in and out of the cells of the body until it is metabolised by enzymes in the liver, which strips it of its methyl groups until it becomes xanthine. The body can use xanthine to make new cellular components; or, if it is not needed, the xanthine can be converted to uric acid and excreted in the urine. The liver can remove any of the methyls from the caffeine molecule, but it tends to remove the one that converts caffeine into paraxanthine, which is more potent than caffeine. This is why the half-life of caffeine in the body is several hours, and why the effect of a cup of coffee can be felt for a long time. (The half-life is the time it takes for the body to reduce the amount of an unnatural chemical by half. After a subsequent half-life it will then be down to a quarter of the original level, then to an eighth, and so on.)

When paraxanthine is again trapped by the enzymes of the liver, a second methyl group is removed and it loses it potency entirely. These processes are slow, and they can be very slow in some people, making their bodies more intolerant of this caffeine. Curiously, the livers of cigarette smokers are much better at metabolising caffeine because of the effect nicotine has on the enzymes, and for these people the half-life of caffeine is much reduced.

Several major investigations have shown that there could be caffeine withdrawal symptoms, and that these consist of headache, depression, fatigue, anxiety irritableness, tense muscles, a jittery feeling, nausea, and even vomiting. As long ago as 1943 it was suggested that those who stopped taking in large amounts of caffeine experienced headaches, which began after two or three days and lasted for about a week. Nor was the effect observed only in those who were heavy users. All these effects are very mild compared to the withdrawal symptoms of other drugs, although some coffee drinkers experience 'cold turkey' symptoms when they stop drinking it. Some people appear to become *addicted* to caffeine, and there is in the US a group calling themselves Caffeine Anonymous.

In fact, caffeine may be viewed in a positive light. It may save lives by keeping drivers awake who might be in danger of nodding off at the wheel. Compared to those other legal drugs, nicotine and alcohol, caffeine appears almost benign. Smoking-related diseases kill around 400 000 in the USA and 100 000 in the UK every year, and alcohol-related diseases and accidents kill around 100 000 in the USA and 25 000 in the UK. Caffeine kills no one.

An alternative menu for those wishing to avoid caffeine is not needed; simply avoid the kinds of foods and drinks on the menu at the start of this chapter.

CHAPTER 7

Sulfur dioxide and sulfites

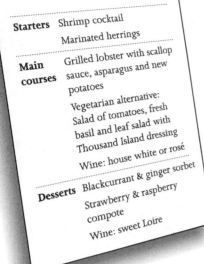

MENU

Starters Shrimp cocktail
Marinated herrings

Main courses Grilled lobster with scallop sauce, asparagus and new potatoes

Vegetarian alternative:
Salad of tomatoes, fresh basil and leaf salad with Thousand Island dressing

Wine: house white or rosé

Desserts Blackcurrant & ginger sorbet
Strawberry & raspberry compote

Wine: sweet Loire

If a group of ten people dined on the above menu, the chances are that by the end of the evening one of them would be suffering the effects of too much sulfur dioxide. That person would soon start wheezing, and they could be well on their way to an attack of asthma. Usually such a person is aware that certain foods will bring on an attack, but many people are only half-aware that they are affected by sulfur dioxide: an encounter with it will leave them a little tight-chested, and wondering if they are starting with a cold. The effect is temporary, and will pass off within a few hours.

A few people are extremely sensitive to sulfur dioxide and for asthmatic patients as little as 1–5 parts per million (p.p.m.) in the air they breathe is enough to trigger an attack. Even normal healthy people will find that inhaling air with 6 p.p.m. of sulfur dioxide will cause breathing difficulties, and this amount of the gas can be present in the air of highly industrialised areas. Asthmatics are much more sensitive to sulfur dioxide because it constricts the airways of the lungs. The 100 mg or so in the food and wine of the above menu would certainly make them very ill.

But it isn't only the sulfur dioxide in food and drink that can affect us, as the case study in the box shows: it can be encountered in many ways. Polluted air in industrial cities, and especially where coal and fuel oil are burnt, can produce levels high enough to affect sensitive people. However, it is in the catering industry that sulfur dioxide is used most, to keep peeled potatoes white and to preserve soft fruits. For these purposes it is sold as a solution in water. In many countries the level of sulfur dioxide in foods and drink is now governed by legislation, although the maximum permitted level in individual foods varies. Wine

Case study: **On a balcony in southern Spain**

Jean was a 42-year-old business woman, with her own company which was very successful. It was based in Gwent, in Wales, and run by a hard-working and trustworthy management team. Indeed, it was doing so well that Jean and her husband decided that they could take long breaks to escape the cold Welsh winters, and so they bought an apartment in the south of Spain. They generally went out there in November to get things ready for their holiday.

Jean took pleasure in decorating and furnishing the apartment, and her final job was to clean the large balcony which was covered with an unsightly black mould. She bought a proprietary cleaner from the local hardware store and began work on it. The day was unpleasantly hot, especially working outside the air-conditioned apartment, but Jean persevered. After two hours she started to have a tight feeling in her chest and throat, but she continued working. Then she collapsed … and woke up the following day in the local hospital's intensive care unit. They thought she had had a heart attack, but over the next few days all the tests showed her to be healthy, and soon she felt perfectly well.

Jean returned home to Wales and decided that part of the trouble was that she was over-weight and unused to physical exercise, and that this—and the hot, sultry weather—had caused her to collapse. She decided to change her life-style, and to help cut down her calorie intake she stopped drinking gin and tonic (her favourite method of relaxing) and began to drink wine and to eat more fresh fruit. She also stopped drinking coffee. A week after her return to Wales she collapsed again, and she ended up in Cardiff Royal Infirmary's intensive care unit. The outcome was the same: 24 hours later she was feeling well again, and tests for heart disease were negative.

A month later it happened a third time, but after that attack she went to a local allergy centre, convinced that she had become allergic to something in her diet. There she was surprised to find herself being questioned about her intake of white wine and fruit drinks. Her change in eating habits had increased greatly her exposure to sulfites and sulfur dioxide. When she was asked about the antifungal cleaner she had used on the balcony in Spain, she remembered that it had a strong sulfur smell. Jean's attacks were all due to sulfur dioxide.

On the advice she was now given she returned to gin and tonic, and stopped taking soft drinks. She was also told which foods to avoid in future. Since that time she has had no recurrence of her symptoms, and she cancelled her follow-up appointment because she now felt that the problem was solved, as indeed it was.

producers cannot do without sulfur dioxide, and other food industries continue to use it because it is a cheap and an effective preservative.

There is no recommended maximum safe daily intake for sulfur dioxide because it is relatively harmless at the levels we encounter it, and if too much were to be used then we would be likely to reject the food and drink containing it because of its unpleasant smell. However, for an unfortunate few it can be hazardous—even deadly—at any level, and it is often undetectable to the human nose and palate.

Sulfur dioxide, sulfites, and food preservatives

The natural background level of sulfur dioxide (SO_2) in the air we breathe has been estimated to be around 3 micrograms (µg) per cubic metre of air, or about 1 part per billion (p.p.b.). Since the Industrial Revolution the level of sulfur dioxide in the Earth's atmosphere has increased greatly, and this is acknowledged in the World Health Organization's recommendation that levels should not exceed 60 µg per cubic metre (20 p.p.b.). Not surprisingly, this level is exceeded at about a third of the sites where it is monitored around the globe. Rural air generally has up to 20 p.p.b. of SO_2, while urban air has about double this, and heavy industrial areas have three times as much.

It is possible that SO_2 in the air is partly to blame for the 'epidemic' of asthma that afflicts so many people in developed nations. But according to a 1993 report by the UK Department of Health's Advisory Group on the Medical Aspects of Air Pollution Episodes, which was headed by Anne Tattersfield, there is no evidence that SO_2 is the reason. The incidence of asthma in children in the former East Germany, where atmospheric pollution by SO_2 was high, was the same as that in West Germany, where levels were much lower.

Sulfur dioxide is manufactured by burning sulfur, in the form of molten droplets of liquid sulfur, in dry air. The reaction gives out a lot of heat, which can be collected by passing the hot sulfur dioxide gas through boilers which turn the waste heat into useful forms of energy. The sulfur for these processes comes from the large amount of sulfur that has to be removed from oil and natural gas before they can be used. Most sulfur dioxide produced industrially goes into the manufacture of sulfuric acid. Some sulfur dioxide is used as a chemical with its own special uses, such as in the manufacture of cellulose and agricultural products. The gas is easily liquefied at −10°C, shipped in pressure vessels, and used in its liquid form. Liquid sulfur dioxide can even be used as a solvent.

Where sulfur dioxide itself is used in food processing, then a solution of the gas in water is generally preferred and is safe to handle. A litre of water will dissolve just under 40 litres of the gas at 20°C, giving a 9–10% solution which is how it is generally sold commercially. This solution is sometimes referred to as sulfurous acid. Even safer to handle are the solid sulfites and metabisulfites, which are the forms most used in food processing. Sulfur dioxide has some useful properties that make it especially attractive to the food industries. It is a preservative and an antioxidant, it prevents browning, it kills bacteria, it can be used as a bleaching agent (for flour), and it stabilises vitamin C. Not surprisingly, it is used in a large variety of foods.

Browning is triggered by an enzyme that used to be known as polyphenol oxidase (PPO), and is now called phenolase. It can oxidise food components such as polyphenols, which then undergo a series of reactions to produce melanins, which are brown. Sulfur dioxide or sulfite solutions will prevent this happening; and they are doubly effective, because not only do they inactivate the phenolase, but they also prevent formation of melanin. (Other anti-browning agents, such as vitamin C (ascorbic acid) work by counteracting the oxidant effect of phenolase with an antioxidant counter-reaction.)

Sulfur dioxide is used on a large scale as a preservative and given the internationally agreed code number 220 (E220 in Europe). The sulfites are given similar numbers, and these are listed in Table 7.1. Which sulfite food additive is used depends on the food itself, but all are treated as 'sulfites' when it comes to analysing them or referring to them in regulations. Sulfites were once used in salad bars to keep fruits and vegetables fresh, but because some people can be badly affected by them, the US Food and Drug Administration banned them. It did not ban sulfites outright, because in certain foods there is no alternative, and they are allowed in dehydrated foods, maraschino cherries, beers, wines, and potatoes. The levels of sulfites vary according to the food in question, and the range is wide: for example, desiccated coconut can have up to 500 p.p.m., whereas dried fruit can have up to 2000 p.p.m. The highest level of all is 30 000 p.p.m., but this is in a rather special case of a technical material, the dried enzyme, papain, which is extracted from papaya.

The world's leading research unit looking into the effects of sulfur dioxide on food is headed by Bronek Wedzicha, a food scientist at the University of Leeds, UK, and author of *Chemistry of Sulfur Dioxide in Foods*. He believes that sulfur dioxide is the most versatile food additive available, and one of the safest. According to Wedzicha, there are many ways in which sulfur dioxide can react with components of our food, but tests on rats have shown that the results of these interactions are safe.

Sulfur dioxide is a reactive chemical, so it is not surprising that it interacts with other components in food. It can do this in two ways: first, as an antioxidant; and secondly as an attacker of other molecules, to which it binds itself. Sulfur dioxide behaves most effectively in this second capacity at acid levels of pH 3–6, the sort of acid conditions that are found naturally in foods. It reacts with various other food components, such as proteins, unsaturated fats, and organic bases. SO_2 also reacts with thiamin (vitamin B_1), rendering it inactive as a vitamin. This is one reason why the use of SO_2 in meat is restricted, because meat can be a key source of this vitamin in our diet. However, SO_2 is permitted in sausages and in the Scottish delicacy, haggis.

Ketone and aldehyde molecules often impart flavour, but by reacting with SO_2 they become involatile and flavourless. In the course of fermentation one particular aldehyde, acetaldehyde, is formed, and this too can react with sulfur dioxide instead of progressing to more oxidised products. The reaction with SO_2 is reversible, and at a later stage the acetaldehyde is released again, which is why many drinks produced by fermenting grape contain this chemical.

Table 7.1 The sulfites used in food.

Sulfite additive	Code number	Also known as ...
Sulfur dioxide	E220	
Sodium sulfite	E221	
Sodium hydrogen sulfite	E222	Sodium bisulfite
Sodium metabisulfite	E223	Disodium disulfite or disodium pyrosulfite
Potassium metabisulfite	E224	Dipotassium disulfite or potassium pyrosulfite
Calcium sulfite	E226	
Calcium hydrogen sulfite	E227	Calcium bisulfite

What's in wine?

In the USA bottles of wine are labelled to warn the drinker that the product contains sulfites. Sulfites were also present in the wines of the ancient world at the time of Christ—from the days of the Roman Empire, and probably even earlier, 'sulfiting' has been a common method of preserving wine. The sulfur dioxide gas was generated by the simple act of burning natural sulfur, and then the grape juice absorbed the fumes. The procedure was very effective, because sulfur dioxide acts as both an antioxidant and a preservative. When the grapes are crushed, the pulp (known as must) is susceptible to oxidation and enzymatic browning caused by acid-forming bacteria, wild yeasts, and moulds. Sulfur dioxide prevents these processes from happening. It is also particularly good at deactivating enzymes in bacteria and wild yeasts: this stops them making use of the sugars from the grapes, and so allows the added cultured yeast to ferment the wine unhindered. Cultured yeasts can survive high levels of sulfur dioxide; indeed, some actually produce more sulfur dioxide themselves from the sulfate that occurs naturally in grapes.

In the Middle Ages vintners in Germany were forced by law to use burning sulfur to cleanse their barrels before filling them with wine, and by the eighteenth century sulfur wicks were used to sterilise the vats and barrels in the best chateaux of Bordeaux. Alternatively sulfite salts could be added to the grape juice, and today vintners add a sulfite solution, or a 6% aqueous solution of SO_2, or even a liquid SO_2 itself. (Home brewers and wine-makers use sulfur dioxide in the form of sodium metabisulfite, better known as campden tablets.) Today there is hardly a wine made anywhere in the world that does not rely on sulfites in one form or another. Wines made without sulfur dioxide or sulfites are rarely a success, and they may have to be pasteurised at some stage to destroy wild yeasts and bacteria. In any case, it is impossible to make entirely sulfite-free wines, because sulfites are produced naturally in wine when the sulfate it contains is reduced to sulfite by the action of enzymes.

The sulfur treatment for wine-making takes place when the grapes are crushed and at the first bottling or during storage, when sulfite is added to stabilise the wine against further unwanted fermentation. Wines may also be treated with more sulfite just before final bottling, to prevent further fermentation, and this might require levels as high as 350 mg per bottle. Using just the right amount of sulfite is part of the vintner's skill.

During the original fermentation stage the level of SO_2 should be around 50–100 p.p.m., while during wine storage it should be around 50–70 p.p.m. The effectiveness of the sulfite depends to a certain extent on the acidity of the wine: the more acidic it is, then the more the sulfite is effective.

Most of the sulfur dioxide eventually reacts with other components in the wine, but some young white wines have noticeable amounts of the gas. However for most people, the residual amount of SO_2 in a glass of wine has no effect. We have the enzymes in our own body to convert sulfite to sulfate, and this joins the substantial quantities of sulfate that are already present in the body, and which we can excrete easily via our urine.

Sulfur dioxide has to be used with care because its aroma is quite unpleasant even at fairly low concentrations, and it is especially unpleasant to some wine tasters who are intolerant of it. The wines most likely to be over-sulfited, which reflects traditional and local customs, are sweet Loire, sweet Bordeaux, and German wines. Most people can smell SO_2 in pure water at a concentration of 11 p.p.m., but in wines its smell is masked, and as much as 100 p.p.m. can be present in a red wine before it is noticed by most drinkers. For white wines the level can be as high as 200 p.p.m., and even then it may not be detectable. In all wines sulfur dioxide is loosely bound to as many as 50 other natural chemicals that are present, and this is what masks its taste: we only smell free SO_2. Regulations that govern sulfites in wines cover both free and chemically bound SO_2, but in red wines the free SO_2 is difficult to measure.

In the second half of the twentieth century the amount of sulfites in wines was much reduced. In 1910 up to 500 p.p.m. was allowed, but by 1990 the maximum permitted was 200 p.p.m., except for sweet wines which were allowed more than this to prevent the extra sugar they contain from being fermented. These changes came about through the activity of food pressure groups, who took up the cudgel on behalf of asthmatics, especially in the USA and Australia, and in both of these wine-producing countries the labels on wines warn either that the product 'contains sulfites' as in the USA, or in Australia that sulfur dioxide has been added. By 1993 the permitted maximum in any kind of Australian wine was 300 p.p.m., and there are pressures to have this reduced even further.

In Europe the maximum permitted levels of total sulfur dioxide in 1993 were 160 p.p.m. in dry red wines, 210 p.p.m. in dry white, dry rosé, and sweet red wines, and 260 p.p.m. in sweet white and rosé wines. (In contrast, the permitted level of sulfur dioxide in beer and cider is 70 p.p.m.) Some wines are permitted to exceed these levels, and sweet white Bordeaux, Jurnaçon, sweet white Loire, Beerenauslese, Tockenbeerenauslese, and Ausbruch wines can have up to 400 p.p.m. It may only be a matter of time before warnings are printed on the labels of European wines, although the tradition of vintage wines will probably make it difficult to enforce. In any event, if a person knows they are intolerant of sulfites, or that they are asthmatic, they should avoid wines and beers, as the case study in the box shows. If they want to drink alcohol, they are best advised to stick to distilled spirits such as vodka and gin, and not to mix these with fruit juices.

Case study: **Only one glass of wine, but one too many**

In 1987 doctors at Tufts Hospital in Boston, USA, described the tragic case of a 33-year-old man who died after drinking a few sips of wine. He had suffered from asthma for nine years, but in 1982 he had a very bad attack after eating a packet of dried apricots, and was rushed to hospital. The next year he had a similar episode after eating salad in a restaurant, and this time he also experienced dizziness and nausea. Again he was hospitalised.

Then in 1985 he suffered a third serious attack which proved fatal. He opened a bottle of dry white wine and after a few sips he collapsed under an immediate and severe attack of asthma. Despite attempts at resuscitation, he died. Analysis of the wine showed that it contained 92 p.p.m. of sulfite (92 mg per litre). In the acidic conditions of the wine this was likely to have been in the form of sulfur dioxide, and even if it were there as sulfite, and so less detectable, when it reached the stomach it would have become SO_2 in the acid conditions that pertain there. Whichever form it was, it triggered spasms in the airways and the release of large amounts of mucous, as was revealed at the post-mortem examination of this unlucky individual.

The effect of sulfur dioxide and sulfites on the lungs and body

Our own bodies produce sulfite quite naturally, during the metabolism of the sulfur-containing amino acids such as cysteine and methionine. Not that our body wants sulfites around—it doesn't, so it removes them quickly by oxidising them to sulfate and excreting them. Most people have more than enough of the necessary enzyme to do this, which is why most people can also cope easily with the sulfites that come as preservatives in the food and drink they consume.

A diagnostic investigation of those who might be sensitive to sulfite is conducted using solutions of potassium metabisulfite. The patient is given these or a placebo, and they swill the solution round their mouth and spit it out. Then their lung function is measured using a technique called total body plethysmography, which can detect changes in the size of the airways. Double-blind testing ensures that the results are valid. If the patient's airways constrict, they are sensitive to sulfite. Then a controlled test is carried out using solutions of increasing strength, starting with 1 mg per litre, and increasing to 200 mg, a value to which anyone will respond who experiences respiratory difficulties. In this way, a threshold sensitivity can be assessed.

Many scientific papers claim that only asthmatics and allergic patients are sensitive to sulfites, but this is not so: it only reflects the crude measures often used to assess sulfite sensitivity. (This topic is discussed in detail in specialist texts such as *Food Allergy* by Dean Metcalfe and colleagues.) But total body plethysmography is a very accurate method of measuring body change, and is used as a research tool by the pharmaceutical industry to detect changes in healthy volunteers. Producing an asthmatic response using sulfite is part of the procedure for testing new anti-asthmatic drugs.

An asthmatic response depends on the fragility of cells that contain biogenic amines such as histamine. These cells can be induced to release their contents, for example in response to a chemical such as SO_2. This process is known medically as degranulation. There are many non-specific triggers for degranulation, such as heat, cold, exercise, smoking, and breathing in chemicals. There is a pharmacological reason for this, which can be demonstrated by the use of atropine, a drug that will block the group of nerves that responds to acetylcholine, and it will block the effects of SO_2 in the airways.

Sulfite sensitivity may also explain why some people suffer from irritable bowel syndrome. Our bodies rely on bacterial fermentation in our intestines to produce some of the simple sugars that we use for energy. Indeed, as much as 25% of the energy we extract from carbohydrate may come by this route. The enzymes in microbes like bacteria break down long-chain sugars, and as they do so they produce various simpler sugars, some of which are important for normal bowel motion. When this goes wrong we may suffer the condition known as irritable bowel syndrome, which is sometimes known as gut fermentation syndrome. The effect is to produce wind and bloating. Sulfites may explain this condition, because of their known ability to suppress some fermentation enzymes while permitting others to operate. Too much sulfite could decrease the numbers of naturally occurring gut microbes, while allowing sulfite-resistant ones to flourish. Tests have shown that those who are sulfite sensitive, and who have a tendency to irritable bowel syndrome, find that this condition responds to a low-sulfite diet.

People who are more susceptible to sulfite are probably lacking in the enzyme sulfite oxidase, which metabolises the active sulfites into inactive sulfates which are then easily excreted. For such people, a sudden intake of sulfite from their diet causes abdominal pain, nausea, and vomiting. Because sulfite is a neurotoxin, it also causes dizziness, lack of co-ordination, and possibly unconsciousness. Other symptoms may be visual disturbance, tremor, and sneezing, all of which can be severe in susceptible individuals, and will appear in milder forms even in normal individuals if enough sulfite is taken into the body.

How much sulfite gets converted to irritating SO_2 depends on whether the local environment is acid or alkali. Food and drink which is particularly acidic, such as white wine and vinegar products, will convert any sulfite to SO_2, and so will the hydrochloric acid in our stomach. Even 5 mg of sulfite in the stomach can be converted to enough SO_2 to trigger an asthmatic attack. In a normal European three-course meal, the amount of sulfite is likely to be 50–100 mg, and a meal chosen from the menu of the start of this chapter, would contain about 100 mg of sulfite.

If you are sensitive to SO_2, you will experience a tight chest when you eat food that has been treated with it. So you should wash all fruit and vegetables, and particularly salads, before you eat them—ideally, you should leave them to soak for a while. The US Food and Drug Administration permits low levels of SO_2 and sulfite to be used in processed, canned, and frozen foods, and provided the total remains below 10 p.p.m. then its presence need not be recorded on the packet or can. This regulation does not apply to wines or beers, and as the amount of SO_2 or sulfite in these drinks may be quite large it is always wise to open the bottle some time before drinking. However, this will only reduce the amount of SO_2 gas dissolved in the drink—it will not affect the level of sulfite.

Here is a list of foods that are commonly sulfited. The list illustrates how difficult it is to calculate how much sulfite we take in each day, because it comes in so many foods:

Pickles	horseradish, pickled onions, relishes, cider vinegar
Seafood	clams, shrimps, lobster, scallops, dried cod
Canned foods	soups, some vegetables, fruits
Vegetables	all processed vegetables
Desserts	jellies, products with gelatin and gums, sweet sauces, toppings, processed yoghurt
Confectionery	baked products containing jams and preserves
Dried foods	bananas, apricots, snacks, soups, desiccated coconut, candied peel

Others   blackcurrant jam, soy protein, seafood pastes, fruit pie fillings, fruit concen-
                  trates, fruit juices, glacé cherries
Drinks   beers, wines, cider

Daunting as this list appears, it is possible to avoid sulfur dioxide and sulfites, even when eating out. The best advice would be to choose a meal from the following menu:

MENU

Starters Sliced melon
Cucumber mousse
and toast

Main courses Fried cod and hand-cut chips with sweetcorn

Vegetarian alternative:
Baked potato with
baked bean filing

Desserts Treacle pudding
and custard

Selection of cheeses

Coffee or tea

CHAPTER 8

Natural toxins

Natural toxins are to be found in all kinds of foods, but they are generally in quantities too tiny to affect us. For example, there is cyanide in almonds and tapioca, hydroxy-tryptamine in cabbages and bananas, and myristicin in nutmeg and carrots. Myristicin can cause hallucinations, but it would be virtually impossible to eat enough carrots to produce the desired effect. On the other hand, nutmeg abuse has been well documented in the medical literature for over a century: a tablespoon of this spice can deliver enough myristicin to cause hallucinations, palpitations, and a feeling of impending doom.

The natural toxins in food fall broadly into two categories: the toxins produced by the degradation of food caused through microorganisms such as viruses, bacteria, fungi, and yeasts; and the toxic chemicals that are an inseparable part of the foods themselves. There are about half a million natural chemicals in the food we eat—a cup of coffee contains around 2000. Only a few of the chemicals in foods have been identified, and even fewer have been tested to see if they are safe; but we eat them and come to no harm. Some non-nutrients in food have been tested and shown to cause cancers in laboratory mice and rats, but they are tested at levels far higher than they occur in our diet. Our body's detoxification system can deal with them easily. Some natural toxins can even occur in the most benign of foods, such as honey—as the box explains.

> ### Mad honey disease
>
> Honey is wholesome and nutritious, but it can make people very ill if it contains a chemical called grayanotoxin. This dangerous honey is made by bees that have collected nectar from rhododendrons, and the illness that follows from eating it is known as rhododendron poisoning or mad honey disease. The condition has been recognised since Roman times and occurs most commonly in Turkey, but has been recorded in the USA. Happily, cases of mad honey disease are extremely rare.

The grayanotoxin affects the receptors in muscle, and especially in heart muscle. It also stimulates the nerves, so that they are switched on but cannot be switched off—they are permanently activated. The toxin binds to a very specific area of the receptor responsible for operating the so-called sodium pump, which generates the electric potential needed to make nerve fibres work.

Those affected by grayanotoxin are in a constant state of activity, which leads to low blood pressure, slowed heart rate, excess salivation, tingling sensations in the skin, and occasionally convulsions. The condition is rarely fatal, but the symptoms need to be treated until the toxic effects gradually wear off; this takes about 24 hours. The characteristic dizziness sometimes starts within minutes of eating the honey, and is followed by weakness, excessive perspiration, nausea, and vomiting, and later by the more serious symptoms of palpitations and breathlessness caused by low blood pressure, a slowing of the heart, and changes in heart rhythm.

Flowers of the rhododendron, azalea, and laurel provide the bees with toxic materials in their nectar, and this will result in contaminated honey. Where these plants are abundant, people should be wary of eating local honey. Turkey and the west coast of America, from British Columbia to California, are the areas where outbreaks of mad honey disease are most likely to occur.

Toxins produced by microorganisms

Most food poisoning is caused by microorganisms (bacteria, protozoa, and viruses): they account for at least 90% of cases. Symptoms appear any time from 12 hours to 10 days after exposure. In the USA, as many as 9000 people die from such causes every year, and half of these deaths are attributed to eating contaminated meat and poultry. The US Centers for Disease Control and Prevention consider the bacteria *Escherichia coli* 0157, *Salmonella*, *Listeria monocytogenes*, and *Campylobacter jejuni* to be of most concern, because of the severity of the illnesses they cause and the frequency of their occurrence. In 1994 in the USA, one outbreak of Salmonella posioning caused by infected ice-cream made 224 000 people ill.

The most likely microorganisms, and the foods most likely to be contaminated are:

Beef	*Escherichia coli* 0157, *Salmonella, Staphylococcus aureus*
Ham and pork	*Salmonella*
Chicken	*Salmonella, Staphylococcus aureus, Campylobacter jejuni*
Eggs	*Salmonella, Staphylococcus aureus*
Cheese	*Escherichia coli, Salmonella*
Fish and shellfish	*Salmonella, Clostridium botulinum, Vibrio cholerae*

Exposure to unfamiliar dangers has increased as world travel has become more common, and as foods from around the world find their way into delicatessens and supermarkets everywhere. The number of serious and fatal incidents caused by food toxins is relatively

low, but for those afflicted the effects are often acute and very debilitating. Alert to the growing danger, the US Food and Drug Administration produced a comprehensive report entitled *Food Borne Pathogenic microorganisms and Natural Toxins* in 1992.

The toxins produced by living organisms in food are classed as either exotoxins or endotoxins. Exotoxins are proteins released by contaminating bacteria, and it is those proteins
that make the micro-organisms dangerous and account for their levels of virulence. Bacteria
divide and multiply rapidly if the conditions are right, and the amount of exotoxin they
secrete likewise increases. If the type of bacteria does not produce an exotoxin then it is generally not as virulent, and we digest the bacteria along with any endotoxins that it may contain. Endotoxins are complex molecules that are an integral part of the structure of
microbial cell walls. Endotoxins can be equally poisonous. The exotoxins are the most
dangerous, but fortunately they are not common. On the other hand, endotoxins are
more common and produce acute symptoms, but they rarely have serious or lasting
consequences.

The exotoxins

Exotoxins have specific biological actions, binding to receptors and blocking essential
metabolic pathways. We have defences against them: they can be broken down by the body's
proteolytic enzymes, which digest protein. The effect in the body will depend on the bacteria and the toxin they produce: enterotoxins attack the gut; neurotoxins attack the nervous
system; leucocidins kill white blood cells; and haemolysins target red blood cells. Other
groups have a broader scatter of shot: For example, *Staphylococcus* and *Streptococcus* produce cytotoxins that breakdown and kill a wide variety of cells.

The really virulent exotoxins are specific to a particular microorganism. For example
botulinum toxin, which is one of the deadliest toxins of all, comes from the bacterium
Clostridium botulinum. As little as 0.8×10^{-8} mg (which is less than a billionth of a gram) is
lethal. The first recorded case of botulinum poisoning was in 1818, but it was not linked to
the toxin until further poisoning occurred as the result of eating raw fish. In Japan and
Alaska, where fish is traditionally eaten raw or lightly cooked, the outbreaks of poisoning
have been more frequent, whereas in the UK and USA this type of poisoning has been
extremely rare, and is almost entirely associated with preserved food products. There were
four deaths in the UK in 1978 as a result of eating canned salmon that had been infected.
Refrigeration may not always be sufficient to prevent organisms from producing exotoxins,
and some, like *Clostridium botulinum*, can withstand cold conditions down to $-5\,^{\circ}$C.

More common contamination comes from various bacteria that can affect fish, and these
can come from the handlers, utensils, and conditions in the premises where the fish is
processed. The commonest organism is *Staphylococcus aureus*, and this is usually the result
of human contamination combined with poor storage temperature control and under-
cooking. *Staphylococcus aureus* affects not only fish, but also other foods that have been
handled by humans: it is sometimes present in the nose, and often present in abscesses, skin
infections, and wounds. Some organisms have been demonstrated to be present even in
frozen food, such as *Listeria* in shrimp and crab.

Table 8. 1 lists the common toxins associated with fish, the food that is most likely to be contaminated. These toxins make us ill in many different ways:

Paralytic shellfish poisoning (PSP) Paralytic shellfish poisoning (PSP) is caused by eating shellfish contaminated with marine algae (dinoflagellates), which are found in latitudes greater than 30° North or South, and where sea temperatures are 15–17 °C. The

Table 8.1 Natural toxins found in fish.

Toxins	Disease	Microorganisms responsible	Clinical features of poisoning
Saxitoxins	paralytic shellfish poisoning (PSP)	*Gonyaulax tamarensis* *Gonyaulax catanella* *Pyrodinium balhamenese*	tingling mouth and extremities, dizziness, floating sensation, paralysis, respiratory distress, death
Brevetoxins	neurotoxic shellfish poisoning (NSP)	*Ptychodiscus brevis*	parasthesae ('pins and needles') abdominal pain, temperature sensations, temporary blindness, paralysis, death
Domoic acid	amnesic shellfish poisoning (ASP)	*Nitzschia pungens*	Nausea, vomiting, disorientation, memory loss, organ failure, death
Okadaic acid Dinophysis toxins Yessotoxin Pectentoxins	diarrhetic shellfish poisoning (DSP)	*Prorocentrum lima* *Dinophysis forti* *Dinophysis acuminata* *Dinophysis norvegica*	Nausea, vomiting diarrhoea, abdominal pain
Ciguatoxin Maltotoxin	ciguatera	*Gambierdiscus toxicus* *Prorocentrum concavum* *Prorocentrum mexicana*	vomiting, diarrhoea dizziness, temperature sensations, temporary blindness, paralysis, death
Tetrodotoxin	puffer fish poisoning	*Vibrio* *Pseudomonas Alteromonas* *Shewanella spp* *Steromones spp*	parasthesae, floating sensation, difficulty swallowing, low blood pressure, slow heart, respiratory distress, ascending paralysis,* death
Tetramine	red whelk poisoning		blurred vision, twitching, weakness, paralysis, collapse
Histamine	scombroid poisoning	*Morganella morganii* *Hafnia alvei,* *Klebsiella pneumoniae* *Proteus spp* *Vibrio spp*	vomiting, diarrhoea burning mouth, flushing rash, low blood pressure, swelling, inflammation

*Ascending paralysis starts at the periphery and works its way centrally as opposed to descending which spreads to the periphery.

algae exist as cysts on the seabed, but given the right conditions they rise to the surface and multiply rapidly, creating so-called red tides. These algal blooms can last for up to three weeks during the summer months, before dying away to be replaced by other algae. Three algae species are linked to PSP: *Gonyaulax catenella* is found along the Pacific coast of North America and in Japan; *Gonyaulax tamarensis* has been associated with outbreaks occurring on the east coast of America and the coast of mainland Europe; and, since the early 1970s, *Pyrodinium balhamenese* has been identified in PSP outbreaks in South America and South East Asia.

In one of the more dramatic incidents, 187 people were ill with PSP in Guatemala in 1987, after eating contaminated local clams; 26 of the people died. In the UK there have been only ten outbreaks of PSP since 1827, and these have been caused by eating mussels. Of the 116 patients affected, 14 have died. The most recent case of PSP recorded in the UK was in 1968, when 78 people became ill after eating mussels fished from the Northumbrian coast that were contaminated with *Gonyaulax tamarensis*. An extensive monitoring programme has since been carried out during high risk periods by the UK Ministry of Agriculture, Fisheries, and Food, involving analysis of coastal waters, shellfish, and crustacea for PSP toxin levels. In 1990, crabs from North Eastern waters were found to contain toxic levels 50 times the acceptable level.

PSP is characterised by numbness in the mouth and fingertips, followed by impaired muscle co-ordination. Respiratory distress and paralysis can occur in severe cases, occasionally with fatal results. The major toxin involved is saxitoxin, which induces paralysis by blocking sodium channels in cell membranes. At least 18 other toxins have been identified, consisting of natural algal toxins, such as neo-saxitoxin produced by *Gonyaulax, tamarensis* var. *excavata*, and metabolised derivatives of algal products found in shellfish. All are heat stable and will survive normal cooking processes. Saxitoxin is one of the most potent poisons known, and listed in Schedule I of the Chemical Weapons Convention. Countries once stockpiled this chemical for military use, but those signing the Convention have had to destroy their stocks and retain just enough for medical research purposes.

Neurotoxic shellfish poisoning (NSP) The toxins that cause neurotoxic shellfish poisoning are produced by the dinoflagellate algae *Ptychodiscus brevis*. Outbreaks of NSP have been associated with the consumption of oysters, clams, and other bivalve molluscs, mainly in North America. *Ptychodiscus brevis* is responsible for Florida's famous red tides, which cause eye irritation and coughs in swimmers exposed to the toxins that are released into the surf by the algae. These are the neurotoxins brevetoxin B and C. The precise mode of action of these polyether molecules is unknown, but they bind to nerve cells and cause gastrointestinal symptoms, numbness of the mouth, muscular aches and dizziness.

Amnesic shellfish poisoning (ASP) Amnesic shellfish poisoning (ASP) was first described in Canada in 1987, when 107 patients were taken ill after eating cultivated blue mussels. Three people died. The symptoms included vomiting, diarrhoea, abdominal cramps, and loss of short term memory, which became permanent in some cases. The chemical responsible was domoic acid from the marine diatom *Nitzschia pungens*, which is widely distributed in the coastal water of the Atlantic, Pacific, and Indian oceans. Domoic acid is a powerful neurotoxin that attacks the central nervous system.

Diarrhetic shellfish poisoning (DSP) Diarrhetic shellfish poisoning (DSP) has been a public health issue in Japan for some time and there have been hundreds of cases in the past 25 years. DSP now has worldwide distribution due to the shifting population patterns of the algae that cause it: *Dinophysis* and *Prorocentrum*. Outbreaks have occurred in the Netherlands, France, and Italy, where 150 people were poisoned by contaminated mussels. Although no cases of DSP have yet been reported in the UK, DSP toxins have been detected in cockles growing in estuary waters.

The major toxins in DSP are okadaic acid and dinophysis toxins 1–3, originally extracted from the blue mussel. Other DSP toxins include yessotoxin and the pectentoxins, which are found in scallops (*Patinopecten yessoensis*). It is possible to destroy the toxin by boiling in water for around 3 hours, but the only real safeguard is to monitor toxic levels in shellfish beds, and to shut these down when high levels are detected. The shellfish most likely to be implicated in DSP are mussels, scallops, and clams. The common symptoms are diarrhoea, vomiting, and abdominal pain, and these can persist for up to three days.

Ciguatera Ciguatera was first documented in the West Indies as long ago as 1555; and in the Pacific in 1606 a Spanish crew, sailing with the explorer de Quiros, suffered its typical gastrointestinal and neurological symptoms. The name ciguatera comes from the marine snail *Turbo pica*, which is called cigua by people living in the Caribbean.

Ciguatera is the most frequently reported food-borne illness associated with a natural toxin. It is also the largest global public health problem associated with seafood: there are 50 000 cases worldwide every year, including 20 000 in the Caribbean. In the USA there are 20 to 30 cases recorded annually by the Centers for Disease Control in Atlanta, but this is only a tiny fraction of the outbreaks. Incidents of ciguatera have even been reported in the UK: the most recent was in 1990, when three people were poisoned when they ate a home-cooked red snapper imported from Oman. The Pacific, Caribbean, and Indian oceans are the danger areas for ciguatera, and the fish involved are mainly the predatory reef fish. Snappers, groupers, jacks, barracudas, surgeon fishes, and sea basses are the main culprits, and over 400 species have been reported as being ciguatoxic.

The symptoms of ciguatera vary widely because several toxins are involved, and the response to each depends on the amount eaten. The clinical features include nausea, vomiting, abdominal pain, dizziness, blurred vision and even blindness (although this may be temporary), sometimes followed by paralysis and death—the mortality rate can be as high as 20%. A curious symptom is the reversal of sensations of heat and cold. These symptoms usually appear within a few hours of eating the fish, but they can appear within 15 minutes or after 24 hours, and the neurological effects can persist for months. There is no antidote to ciguatoxin: treatment is supportive, and certain foods, such as alcohol, fish, nuts and nut oils, should be avoided during the recovery period as they exacerbate the symptoms.

It was only in 1977 that the origin of ciguatera poisoning was discovered to be the algae *Gambierdiscus toxicus*. Two other algae, *Prorocentrum concavum* and *Prorocentrum mexicana*, produce similar neurotoxins. Ciguatoxins are low molecular weight polyethers that play havoc with the body's neurotransmitters by attaching themselves to nerve endings and disrupting the release of essential messenger chemicals.

Ciguatoxins are unaffected by cooking and processing, and contaminated fish look normal. The only advice available to consumers is to avoid large fish of the hazardous species, because these will have the greatest concentration of the toxins. The recent development of methods of immunoassay, including a dip-stick test, has helped to reduce the dangers by facilitating the monitoring of high-risk locations.

Puffer fish poisoning Incidents of puffer fish poisoning are rare outside Japan, but there have been more than 6000 cases there this century. Such is the threat it poses that puffer fish chefs have to be licenced in Japan, and even so the Constitution forbids the Emperor from eating this delicacy.

The symptoms are numbness in the face and extremities, a floating sensation, weakness, ascending paralysis, and respiratory failure. The disease has a mortality rate approaching 60%. Onset is usually within three hours, and symptoms may last for three days—provided the patient survives the first 24 hours.

The toxins in puffer fish are tetrodotoxin and its derivative anhydrotetrodotoxin, which are concentrated in the skin and viscera of puffer fish, porcupine fish, and ocean sunfish. They block one of the sodium channels, the fast channel, through cell membranes. Tetrodotoxin may have a bacterial origin—bacteria belonging to *Vibrio spp*, *Shewanella spp*, *Pseudomonas spp*, and *Steromonas spp* have been shown to produce it. Tetrodotoxin is not destroyed by cooking.

Red whelk poisoning Six incidents of red whelk poisoning have been recorded in the UK since 1970—four in Scotland and two in the North of England. All followed consumption of red whelk (*Neptunea antoqua*), which is occasionally caught by fishermen trawling for edible whelk (*Buccinium undatum*) off the north-east coast of Britain. These whelks look similar, but the red whelk is larger and smoother than the edible whelk and is a yellow/orange colour. The red whelk contains the metabolite tetramine in its salivary gland, and it is this curare-like compound that acts as the poison. It affects the nervous system, producing blurred vision, muscular twitching, weakness, paralysis, and collapse. The symptoms tend to disappear within 24 hours.

Scombroid fish poisoning Scombroid fish poisoning is caused by the release of histamine, and is dealt with in Chapter 4.

The endotoxins

Endotoxins are a combination of fat (lipo) and carbohydrate (saccharide) molecules, and are called lipopolysaccharides. They are particularly associated with Gram-negative bacteria (see the Glossary). They tend to be less potent than the exotoxins, and because they come from the breakdown products of the bacterial cell wall, the toxic reaction is directly linked to the quantity of endotoxin released and produces less specific symptoms (fever, joint pains, diarrhoea, and vomiting) and they do not interfere with receptors, or target one organ system. However, unlike some of the exotoxins, they are heat-resistant; this means that while cooking contaminated food may kill the bacteria, it won't rexmove the toxins that can cause acute illness. It is for this reason that reheated foods, in which the bacteria have been multiplying, are often to blame for endotoxic poisoning. The effects come on rapidly after a few hours and usually consist of severe vomiting, followed by abdominal cramps and diarrhoea. Fortunately, these symptoms are short-lived and clear up within a day.

However, if live bacteria leave the gut and invade the body, major problems arise. This can happen if the body is severely compromised by starvation or disease, for then the bacteria may be able to overcome the body's defences and enter the tissues. As the invading bacteria increase in numbers and die, they cast off massive amounts of endotoxin. This larger dose of toxin causes more severe symptoms such as fever, shock, and collapse. It can sometimes restrict the flow of blood around the body, starving key organs, with fatal consequences.

Poisoning by endotoxins this rarely happens with food kept in hygienic conditions. Indeed, good hygiene is the best defence against endotoxins and failure to observe any of the following advice could put your health, the health of your family, or your business, at risk.

Human factors

- Wash hands before food preparation
- Wash hands regularly during food preparation
- Cover any wounds
- Do not sneeze or cough over food, and if you have a cold, wear a mask
- Keep hair covered
- Wear clean clothes

Preparation area

- Keep the preparation area clean, and do not work on damaged surfaces
- Keep perishable foods in a refrigerator when not in use
- Keep uncooked foods cool and in the dark
- Keep pets and animals out the cooking area

Utensils

- Do not use a cutting board that can not be sanitized
- Sanitize cutting tools before use
- Sanitize cutting tools used on raw foods before using them on cooked foods
- Keep utensils clean, and store them in a clean area

Food

- Wash thoroughly all fresh vegetables and fruit
- Throw away contaminated food
- Do not use food that has deteriorated
- Do not use food from damaged cans or packages
- If something smells wrong, throw it away
- Do not keep raw food close to, or above, cooked foods in a refrigerator

Cooking

- The minimum cooking temperature for beef should be 60 °C (140 °F); for pork, veal, and lamb it should be 77 °C (170 °F) and for turkey and all poultry it should be 82 °C (180 °F)
- For large joints and fowl, check the temperature of the meat with a cook's thermometer

- Use a microwave oven for full defrosting before cooking
- Take special care when cooking dishes that use low temperatures and slow cooking

It should always be borne in mind that any food may be contaminated, so it should always be cleaned thoroughly, stored under the right conditions, and cooked correctly. Failure to follow these simple guidelines explains the ever-increasing numbers of food-poisoning outbreaks in developed countries like the UK.

Naturally occurring plant poisons

Throughout the plant and animal kingdoms there are numerous chemicals that are poisonous to humans, and these are usually well known, easily identified, and thereby avoided. However, there are some which represent hidden dangers in food, and the remainder of this chapter will deal with these.

Mushroom toxins

Mushrooms are a highly esteemed food, and it is only the fear of being poisoned that limits most people's consumption to the common cultivated mushroom (*Agaricus bisporus*). This course of action was encouraged in medieval times by monks, although they realised that there was a host of other delicious, and edible, fungi. They also knew that there were several very poisonous ones, so they encouraged the peasantry to stick to the common mushroom for safety. It has been suggested that there was a hidden agenda behind this advice: it left the better-tasting mushrooms for the monks. This fear of unusual mushrooms continues to the present day, but it is now giving way to a more enlightened view of edible fungi, as people realise that other varieties are often consumed in other cultures.

The commonly eaten fungi are the oyster mushroom (*Pleurotus ostreatus*), the padi-straw mushroom of East Asia (*Volvariella volvaceae*), the shiitake of Japan (*Lentinus edodes*), and the truffles (*Tuber melanosporum/magnatum*) and chanterelles (*Cantharellus cibarius*) of France. These are now appearing on supermarket shelves around the world. The larger meatier field mushroom (*Agaricus campestris*), although edible, does not lend itself to commercial production. The world's biggest producers of mushrooms are the USA, France, Taiwan, and the UK, in that order, with a total world production of 1 000 000 tons per annum. In the UK mushroom production is a £200 000 000-a-year business.

There are dangers in eating the wrong fungi, and while only a few contain deadly poisons, many can cause acute unpleasant effects. The severity of mushroom poisoning, and its outcome, depends on the quantity of mushrooms consumed. It is not always possible to identify the poisons, and for this reason they are categorised by the physiological changes they produce. There are four different types: protoplasmic poisons, which kill cells throughout the body, resulting in organ failure; neurotoxins, which produce neurological symptoms such as profuse sweating, coma, convulsions, hallucinations, excitement, depression, and spasms in the gut; gastrointestinal irritants, with the rapid onset of nausea, followed by vomiting, abdominal cramps, and diarrhoea; and disulfram toxins, whose unpleasant symptoms only appear if alcohol is consumed within 72 hours, when the result is nausea, vomiting and abdominal cramps.

Protoplasmic poisons Several mushroom species, including the death cap or destroying angel (*Amanita phalloides, Amanita virosa*) and the fool's mushroom and some of its relatives, produce a family of poisonous cyclic octapeptides called amanitins. Poisoning is characterized by a long latent period (up to 48 hours in some cases, although the average is 6–15 hours) during which the patient shows no symptoms. Then there are sudden, severe seizures of abdominal pain, persistent vomiting and watery diarrhoea, extreme thirst, and lack of urine production. If the patient survives this early phase, he or she may appear to recover for a short time, but this period will generally be followed by a rapid and severe loss of strength, prostration, and pain-caused restlessness. Death occurs in 50–90% of cases, due to progressive and irreversible kidney, liver, and skeletal muscle damage, and may follow within 48 hours of eating a large helping of the mushrooms. More typically the disease lasts 6–8 days in adults, and 4–6 days in children. Two or three days after onset jaundice, cyanosis, and coldness of the skin can occur, and death usually follows a period of coma and occasionally convulsions. (If the patient survives all this, they generally require at least a month to recover, and there is still some enlargement of the liver.) Autopsy will usually reveal fatty degeneration and necrosis of the liver and kidney.

Certain species of false morel (*Gyromitra esulenta* and *Gyromitra gigas*) contain the protoplasmic poison gyromitrin, a volatile hydrazine derivative. Poisoning by this toxin superficially resembles the poisoning described above but it is less severe. There is generally a latent period of 6–10 hours after ingestion during which no symptoms are evident, followed by sudden onset of abdominal discomfort (a feeling of fullness), severe headache, vomiting, and sometimes diarrhoea. The toxin affects primarily the liver, but there are additional disturbances to blood cells and the central nervous system. The mortality rate is relatively low (2–4%).

Poisonings with symptoms almost identical to those produced by *Gyromitra* have also been reported after ingestion of early false morel (*Verpa bohemica*). Its toxin is presumed to be related to gyromitrin, but has yet to be identified.

The third type of protoplasmic poisoning is caused by the sorrel webcap mushroom (*Cortinarius orelanus*) and some of its relatives. This mushroom produces orellanine, and the poisoning has an extremely long latent period of 3–14 days during which no symptoms are manifest. The first signs are an intense burning thirst (polydipsia) and excessive urination (polyuria). This may be followed by nausea, headache, muscular pains, chills, spasms, and loss of consciousness. In severe cases, renal tubular necrosis and kidney failure may result in death several weeks after the poisoning. There is also fatty degeneration of the liver and severe inflammatory changes in the intestine, and recovery in less severe cases may take several months.

Neurotoxins Neurotoxins attack the nervous system. The symptoms they cause fall into three distinct groups, and the illnesses are named according to the substances responsible for these symptoms.

Muscarine poisoning Ingestion of onocybe or clitocybe species (such as *Onocybe geophylla* or *Clitocybe dealbata*) results in an illness characterized primarily by profuse sweating. This effect is caused by high levels (3–4%) of muscarine, and poisoning by this natural toxin also produces increased salivation and a copious flow of tears, which start within 15–30 minutes after the mushrooms have been eaten. With large doses, these symptoms may be followed by abdominal pain, severe nausea, diarrhoea, blurred vision, and laboured breathing. Symptoms generally subside within two hours and death is rare, but may result from cardiac or respiratory failure in severe cases.

Ibotenic acid and muscimol poisoning   The fly agaric mushroom (*Amanita muscaria*) and panther cap mushroom (*Amanita pantherina*) both produce ibotenic acid and muscimol. These substances produce the same effects, but muscimol is five times more potent than ibotenic acid. Symptoms of poisoning generally occur within 1–2 hours of eating the mushrooms. An initial abdominal discomfort may be present or absent, but the chief symptoms are drowsiness and dizziness (sometimes accompanied by sleep), followed by a period of hyperactivity, excitability, illusions, and delirium. Periods of drowsiness may alternate with periods of excitement, but symptoms generally fade within a few hours. Consumption of large quantities of these mushrooms may cause convulsions, coma, and other neurological problems for up to 12 hours. Fatalities rarely occur in adults, but children are more vulnerable.

Psilocybin poisoning   A number of mushrooms belong to the genera *Psilocybe, Panaeolus, Copelandia, Gymnopilus, Conocybe* and *Pluteus*. When ingested, they produce a syndrome similar to alcohol intoxication (sometimes accompanied by hallucinations). Several of these mushrooms (such as *Psilocybe cubensis, Psilocybe mexicana,* and *Conocybe cyanopus*) are deliberately eaten for their psychotropic effects in religious ceremonies by certain native Americans. The toxic effects are caused by psilocin and psilocybin.

Symptoms usually begin rapidly and generally subside within two hours. Poisonings by these mushrooms are rarely fatal in adults, and may be distinguished from ibotenic acid poisoning by the absence of drowsiness or coma. The most severe cases of psilocybin poisoning occur in small children, where large doses may cause hallucinations accompanied by fever, convulsions, coma, and death. These mushrooms are generally small, brown, nondescript, and not particularly fleshy; they are seldom mistaken for food fungi by hunters of wild mushrooms.

Poisonings caused by eating these mushrooms must be handled with care. The only cases likely to be seen by a physician are those caused by a combination of the mushrooms and some other psychotropic substance such as the designer drug PCP (Angel Dust).

Gastrointestinal irritants numerous mushrooms, including the green gill
(*Chlorophyllum molybdites*), gray pink gill (*Entoloma lividum*), tigertop (*Tricholoma pardinum*), Jack O'Lantern (*Omphalotus illudens*), naked brimcap (*Paxillus involutus*), sickener (*Russula emetica*), early false morel (*Verpa bohemica*), horse mushroom (*Agaricus arvensis*), and pepper bolete (*Boletus piperatus*), contain toxins that can cause gastrointestinal distress, including nausea, vomiting, diarrhoea, and abdominal cramps. In many ways these symptoms are similar to those caused by the deadly protoplasmic poisons. The chief and diagnostic

difference is that poisoning by these mushrooms comes on quickly, rather than the delayed onset seen in protoplasmic poisonings.

Some mushrooms, including the first five species mentioned above, may cause vomiting and/or diarrhoea that last for several days. Fatalities caused by these mushrooms are relatively rare, and are associated with dehydration and electrolyte imbalances resulting from the diarrhoea and vomiting, especially in debilitated, very young, or very old patients. Replacements of fluids and other appropriate supportive therapy will prevent death in these cases. The metabolic chemistry of the toxins responsible for this type of poisoning is still not understood, but it may be related to the presence in some mushrooms of unusual sugars and amino acids.

Disulfiram–like poisoning The ink cap mushroom (*Coprinus atramentarius*) is most commonly responsible for disulfiram-like poisoning, although a few other species have also been implicated. A complicating factor is that this species is generally considered edible, and illness only results when alcoholic beverages are taken at the same time. The mushroom produces an unusual amino acid, coprine, which is converted to cyclopropanone hydrate in the human body. This compound interferes with the detoxification of alcohol, and consumption of alcoholic beverages within 72 hours after eating it will cause headache, nausea, vomiting, flushing, and cardiovascular disturbances that last for 2–3 hours—just as occurs when Antabuse (disulfiram) is taken as a treatment for alcoholism, as described in Chapter 2.

Mould toxins

Moulds are a type of fungi, but unlike mushrooms they are not used as a food. However, they can contaminate foods, and they produce toxins, called mycotoxins, of various types. An outstanding example is the mould *Claviceps purpurea*, a black sclerotic species that produces ergot, a mycotoxin that is also a potent drug, and which is used for the treatment of migraine. The active ingredients of ergot are alkaloids, and rye is deliberately grown in this contaminated state in order to extract and purify these chemicals for use in medicine. *Claviceps purpurea* grows on cereals, particularly rye, contaminating the seed head, and when the cereal is harvested the mould is gathered with the grain. If the grain is fed to animals, acute severe poisoning results; and if it is milled, the flour is then dangerous to humans.

In the Middle Ages, in regions such as the Balkans where rye bread was a common commodity, there were often outbreaks of ergot posioning. The disease was known as St Anthony's fire because it produced a burning sensation in the limbs due to constriction of the blood vessels, which eventually led to gangrene. Convulsions, spasms in the limbs, and death were common. One outbreak occurred in Russia in August 1722, when Peter the Great was poised to begin his great campaign to drive the Turks from Russian soil. His army had assembled at Astrakhan on the delta of the Volga, and was being fed with local rye, which was badly infected with *Claviceps purpurea*. So many men and horses went down with mycotoxin poisoning and died, that the campaign had to be abandoned without a battle being fought.

Other moulds produce other mycotoxins. In 1959 a farmer bought some ground-nut meal to feed to his chickens, and growing on the meal was the powdery green mould

Aspergillus flavus. The chickens ate the meal, and soon they were all dead. This incident led to the research that uncovered a dangerous chemical, the mycotoxin called aflatoxin, in *Aspergillus flavus* and other moulds.

There are four types of aflatoxin—B_1, B_2, G_1, and G_2—with B_1 being the most potent. The foods commonly associated with aflatoxin contamination are corn, peanuts, cottonseed, tree nuts like Brazil, pecan, pistachio, and walnuts, chillies, dried fruit, and even bread, but rarely at levels that our body's detoxification mechanism can not cope with. Cows that have been fed aflatoxin-contaminated feed not only excrete aflatoxin in their urine, but it can also be detected in their milk. Legislation now limits the amount of aflatoxin that is permitted in milk for human consumption, and the European Union has set limits for the aflatoxin B_1 content of animal feed at 20–50 µg per kilogram of feed. If foods like peanuts are found to exceed such levels, they are regarded as unfit for humans.

Aflatoxin poisoning is rare in developed countries, but outbreaks have occurred in Turkey and Kenya. In 1974 in north-west India an outbreak hit two nearby villages, which affected 397 people and left 108 dead. The explanation was contaminated corn, and it caused fever, jaundice, swelling of the legs, pain, and ultimately liver failure. Dogs in the villages died as well. Ten years later the survivors were re-examined by the authorities and found to be completely recovered with no evidence of long-lasting effects. Cirrhosis in children in India correlates with a high intake of crude peanut oil and par-boiled rice, which may have aflatoxin levels of 0.1 mg per kilogram.

A liver cancer that is common in developing countries in East Africa, the Philippines, and Thailand has been epidemiologically linked to aflatoxins, but whether these really are the cause is still debated. However, aflatoxins are known to cause cancer in rats, and so they are used in tests for anticancer drugs. For example, recent research has revealed there is a natural component of certain green vegetables that might prevent tumours from forming; and it has been shown to be effective in rats fed high levels of the most dangerous form of aflatoxin. This natural anticancer agent is indole-3-carbinol (I3C) and it is a component of vegetables such as Brussels sprouts and broccoli. Maggie Manson, Ann Hudson, and colleagues, at the Medical Research Council Toxicology Unit at Leicester University, England, fed I3C to rats that have been given relatively large amounts of aflatoxin B_1 for much of their life, and they failed to develop liver cancer. Tests on a group of rats fed 2 p.p.m. of aflatoxin in their diet for 24 weeks showed an average of six tumours per animal at the end of 48 weeks. A second group put first on a diet rich in I3C for two weeks, and then fed both I3C and aflatoxin B_1, for 22 weeks, developed no tumours after 48 weeks. A more aggressive regime involved feeding a third group aflatoxin B_1, for 6 weeks, then adding I3C to their diet, but continuing with aflatoxin for a further 18 weeks. Even so, no tumours were detected in the rats at the end of their 48-week lifespan either.

Other mycotoxins that may cause disease are listed in Table 8.2. They can be quite resistant to cool temperatures, and storage is therefore of paramount importance, but moulds do not thrive when the moisture content is low, and foods with less than 12% water content are generally regarded safe. But not all moulds are our enemies: some bring great benefits, and these are listed in Table 8.3.

Table 8.2 Mycotoxins in food.

Mycotoxin	Organisim	Foods involved	Disease
Citrinin	*Penicillium citrinum/ viridicatum*	wheat, rye, oats, rice, cheese	kidney damage
Ochratoxins	*Aspergillus ochraceus Penicillium viridicatum*	cereals, coffee, cocoa, citrus fruit, nuts, cheese, soya	fatty liver
Penicillic acid	*Penicillium cyclopium Penicillium martensii*	beans, corn, fruit	liver cancer
Sterigmatocystin	*Aspergillus versicolor*	green coffee, cheese, cereals	liver damage, liver cancer
Trichothecenes	*Fusarium graminearum*	cereals	alimentary tract aleukia
Zearalenone	*Fusarium graminearum*	cereals	oestrogenic hormone mimic

Table 8.3 Beneficial moulds.

Organism	Effects	Product
Saccharomyces cerevisiae	ferments sugars	alcohol
Saccharomyces carlesburgii	ferments sugars	lager
Aspergillus soyae/oryyzae	ferments soya	soy sauce
Penicillium notatum	produces antibiotic	penicillin
Streptomyces griseus	produces antibiotic	streptomycin
Penicillium roquefortii	ripens cheese	Roquefort/Stilton/Gorgonzola
Penicillium camembertii	ripens soft cheese	Camembert and Brie
Mucor/Rhizopus	modifies rice	ragi
Saccharomyces sake	ferments rice	sake
Rhizopus oligosporus	modifies/ferments soya	tempeh
Fusarium graminearum	modifies base foods	Quorn high-protein meat substitute
Aspergillus niger	ferments sugar	citric acid, soft drinks

Pyrrolizidine alkaloids

Pyrrolizidine alkaloids (PAs) are insidious natural toxins. They not only cause the usual symptoms of an overloaded detoxification mechanism, such as diarrhoea and vomiting, but are also capable of causing cirrhosis of the liver, when taken over a long period. Moreover, tests on laboratory mich have shown PAs to be potent carcinogens and mutagens, in other words they can cause cancer and harm embryos. Yet comfrey, a herb rich in PAs, was once commonly used: the leaves of the plant were added to salads, or they were dried and used to make comfrey tea. Practitioners of herbal medicine sold comfrey capsules for those who belived the old lore that comfrey was good for arthritis, headaches, and common colds. Comfrey is now banned for human consumption in Europe, but grazing animals may still be exposed to PAs if they eat ragwort, which also has very high levels. Comfrey and ragwort are both from the *Boraginacae* family of plants, many members of which, including borage, forget-me-not, worts, and hound tongue, contain PAS, as does the *Compositae* family, which includes the daisy, marigold, chamomile, ragweed, heliotrope, groundsel, thistles, and cornflowers. The *Leguminosae* family, which includes the pod-producing beans, is also frequently incriminated.

There are more that a hundred different PAs, and it is difficult to identify the exact one that is responsible for a particular response. They can be consumed in cereals, where the grain has become contaminated with other plant material. Contamination of animal feed may result in milk being affected. But the commonest cause of PA poisoning in the western world is the use of herbal teas and home remedies.

The clinical findings are similar to Budd–Chiari syndrome, a disease in which the vein leaving the liver becomes blocked, causing the liver to swell up. This produces an increased pressure, and large amounts of fluid are forced back into the abdominal cavity—a condition known as ascites. Pyrrolizidine alkaloids produce a similar picture with abdominal pain and nausea, and abdominal distention with prominent dilated vessels on the abdominal wall. Investigations reveal liver damage; and sometimes the lungs are affected, which can be fatal. Low doses of PAs, ingested over a period of time, lead to a different type of liver damage causing fibrosis, which is indistinguishable from cirrhosis. Cirrhosis develops slowly over many years. To begin with the liver fills with fats and enlarges, then fibrosis sets in, when, as its name suggests, the liver becomes fibrous. At this stage the liver starts to shrink and the condition is now called cirrhosis.

One woman who consumed a large amount of herbal tea made from comfrey was diagnosed as having liver damage, and this was still in evidence two years later. Another woman returning to the USA from Ecuador developed severe liver failure with massive ascites, and it transpired that she had been drinking a herbal tea for six months. She was checked one year after she had stopped drinking the tea, and her liver function was back to normal. Two children who were mistakely given *Senecio longibilis* in a Mexican herbal tea called 'gordolobo yerba' were also posioned by PAs. The first child died 8 days later of acute liver failure; the second recovered, but was found six months later to have extensive fibrosis progressing to cirrhosis.

Cyanogens

Cyanogens are sugar molecules, mainly glucose, to which there is attached a cyanide group (chemcial formula CN). Foods which contain cyanogens can be made edible by mixing with water, which enables glucosidase enzymes to work on these toxins, releasing the cyanide as hydrogen cyanide (HCN) which is volatile, so that subsequent heating will expel it. Cyanogens are present in lima beans, cassava, sorghum, etc. as well as in apple pips, and the stones of plums, prunes, apricots, and peaches.

The cyanogens, and the chemically related thiocyanates, are toxic, and they can be fatal in small doses. When consumed in less-than-fatal doses, they produce a range of symptoms. The commonest source of cyanogens is cassava, a small tropical shrub that has edible roots that are used to make flour, or eaten as a vegetable, or made into tapioca. Its leaves are also edible, and contain more nutrients than the roots.

Cassava originated in Brazil, and was transported to Africa by the Portuguese in the sixteenth century. Its importance as a crop can be judged from its ranking as the third among the vegetable crops of the world. Leading producers are Nigeria, Brazil, Thailand, Zaire, and Indonesia, which together produce 157 000 000 metric tons per year and it is a staple food for an estimated 500 million people. A small amount is grown in the southern USA. Cassava is a very nutritions food: it is good source of protein, calcium, phosphorus, iron, and vitamins A, C, and most of the Bs (though not B_{12}); it is also very rich in carbohydrate. However, it also provides cyanogens, and so requires special preparation.

Cyanogen poisoning is most common in those African countries where cassava is part of the staple diet. The toxin in the root is linamarin, which is metabolised in humans to form cyanide, so cassava must never be eaten raw—mostly it is peeled and cooked in water before being eaten. The method of cassava fermentation that people in West Africa practise converts the cyanogenic toxins to volatile hydrogen cyanide using the cassava's own enzymes. The Alur tribe to Uganda are able to reduce cyanogen levels from 400 to 20 mg per kilogram. There is no reduction in the nutritional value of the food.

In the human body, the small amount of cyanide that is present in many foods, notably the brassicas, such as cabbages and turnips is detoxified by being converted to thiocyanate (SCN^-). High levels of thiocyanate however, interfere with iodine metabolism and with the uptake of iodine by the thyroid gland. A study of women in Tanzania showed that those who ate cassava as their staple food had an incidence of goitre, a disease of iodine deficiency, of 73%. Research showed that mechanical milling could reduce the thiocyanate content of cassava, and once this process was introduced the number of people with goitre dropped dramatically.

Konzo: the disease caused by cyanide in food

Cases of konzo were first reported in the 1930s, and the name, which means 'tied legs' derived from the condition of its victims, who were unable to walk. While most recovered after a few days, some were left permanently paralysed. The cause was unknown. In the 1980s many more cases were reported in the drought-affected and war-torn regions of Africa, such as Mozambique, Tanzania, Zaire, and the Central African Republic. For a while doctors thought they were dealing with a new infectious disease, and dismissed the popular belief that it was caused by eating cassava, because the symptoms were not those of cyanide poisoning. If konzo was caused by an infection, this would explain why whole families and villages could be affected while neighbouring areas were free of the disease.

The answer was that konzo came as a result of chronic cyanide poisoning, and often occurred when people began to eat cassava for the first time, but who were unfamiliar with the ways in which it should be prepared so as to remove most of the cyanide it contains. In East Africa the appearance of konzo coincided with the opening of a tarmac road in 1974. This facilitated the transport of cassava into the region and its cheapness encouraged peasant families to start eating it, and then growing it for themselves, especially when they realised that it would produce high yields in poor soil and under drought conditions. Moreover, the cassava roots are protected by the cyanogens, which are natural pesticides, and they also deter hungry monkeys from eating them since they taste so bitter.

It is the more bitter forms of cassava which have the higher levels of linamarin. A kilogram of such cassava, which is equivalent to two fresh roots, can contain enough of the natural toxin to release 1000 mg of cyanide, and this is more than ten times the fatal dose. Grating, and soaking the roots for several days, will release the cyanide in the form of HCN which is then poured off with the water if the cassava is to be dried to make flour, or which boils off if the vegetable is then cooked. The World Health Organisation recommends a maximum level of cyanide in cassava flour of 10 mg per kg.

Konzo mainly appeared in the dry season when there was a high consumption of cassava that had been badly processed. The condition was exacerbated in times of drought and starvation when there was also a shortage of protein. Protein supplies the body with the sulfur-containing amino acids, such as methionine, that it needs to convert the cyanide to thiocyanate, and so detoxify it. Those suffering from *konzo* excrete 10–20 times as much thiocyanate in their urine compared to healthy individuals.

Psoralens

Psoralens are natural insecticides produced by some plants. They have an unusual toxicity in that they sensitize people to light and induce a dermatitis among those who handle foods that contain them, and both may also happen to those sensitive individuals who eat such foods. They are found particularly in celery, and recently a new cultivar that had been developed to be more pest-resistant was responsible for a sudden increase in dermatitis in grocery workers. Because psoralen is a natural insecticide, it is not regulated, and consequently this dermatitis continues to occur in workers handling celery. People who eat celery are not exposed to enough to affect them.

There are other compounds with similar properties, such as bergapten and xanthotoxin, and these are found in a number of other foods, including dill, fennel, angelica, parsley, bergamot, mustard, parsnips, fig, and lime. In 1995 the Burns Center in Brussels reported four cases of partial skin burns after contact with parsley, where psoralen levels had increased due to spoilage. It is essential to be careful when handling any of these plants in any quantity.

Solanine and chaconine

Solanine is a natural toxin that is most commonly associated with the potato. This is not the only food to have high levels of it, but the potato is most likely to be the cause of solanine poisoning.

Solanine is a glyco-alkaloid consiting of a carbohydrate component (the glyco part) and a chemical called solanidine (the alkaloid part). The chemically related alkaloids chaconine and tomatidine, as well as solanine, are found in green peppers, chillies, tomato, and eggplants (aubergines). Poisoning from these vegetable is not reported extensively, though one group did suffer severe effects after competing in a chilli-eating contest, where, perhaps not surprisingly, the symptoms were almost exclusively gastrointestinal. The capsacin, the chemical which gives chillies their firey taste, is also a close relative of solanine.

Proving that solanine has caused food poisoning may not be easy, as the following story illustrates. It was published in the *Quarterly Journal of Medicine*, in 1979, by Mary McMillan and James Thompson, and it is worth recounting in detail.

The story is set in a boys' school in South East London. It was early September in 1969, and the second day of term. Many of the 300 pupils, aged between 11 and 15, stayed to lunch in the school, and that day the main course consisted of meat pie, gravy, boiled potatoes, and greens. Afternoon classes passed off normally, but by 8 o'clock that evening many of the boys were ill with diarrhoea and vomiting, which became progressively worse as the evening wore on. In total 78 boys were affected, 17 of them required hospital admission, and three were dangerously ill. But the majority of boys who had eaten the midday meal at school had not been taken ill. No boys were to be affected in the days that followed, nor were any members of the sick boys' families taken ill in the same way.

It would have been easy to dismiss the incident as an outbreak of food poisoning, but because three boys were extremely ill it was necessary to carry out a thorough investigation as to the cause. The hospital records showed how serious some of the cases were. For example:

S.M. became restless and delirious 20 hours after eating his midday meal. On admission he was unconscious, responding only to painful stimuli, and was extremely restless with ashen faces. Temperature 37.5 °C; pulse rate 160 per minute, and very weak, and respiration 48 per minute; blood pressure unrecordable.

For 24 hours 'S.M.' had a high fever, yet his hands and feet remained cold. In the next 24 hours his circulatory condition slowly improved, but he remained semi-conscious and restless. The pupils of his eyes were small, but they dilated widely from time to time, and yet they were not responsive to light. On the third day he began to talk excessively and nonsensically, he was still very restless, and at times he hallucinated. On the fourth day he showed signs of improving, and by the fifth day he was talking normally and was clearly on the way to recovery.

The three boys most dangerously ill were treated with hydrocortisone, to counter the physical symptoms, paraldehyde to sedate them, and diazepam to reduce anxiety. They were also given the antibiotic chloramphenicol as a precaution, but this was discontinued when it was clear that they were not suffering from a salmonella infection. These boys, and five others who continued to vomit, became moderately dehydrated, and were given fluids intravenously.

All the hospitalized boys were well enough to go home within six to eleven days of admission, and when examined four or five weeks later there was no evidence of long-term effects. Shortly after being discharged, one boy complained of blurred vision, another of giddiness, yet another visual disturbances, and 'S.M.' experienced calf pain on walking. All these symptoms were transient. Another boy had desquamation, the technical term for shedding skin, which occurred from his hands and feet, and there were scars on his legs and buttocks due to spots.

At the invitation of the local Medical Officer of Health, a group of experts visited the school soon after the outbreak, and they quickly realised that they were not dealing with a simple outbreak of food poisoning. The kitchen equipment at the school was inspected and the food hygiene standards could not be faulted. All the boys had eaten the same meal. So what could have caused such different reactions? Why had most boys who had eaten lunch that day not been affected?

The only component of the midday meal that was common to all who were taken ill was the potatoes. One boy who was affected was a vegetarian, which ruled out the meat pie and gravy as the cause, and many of the boys did not eat the green vegetables that were on offer. Yet the teachers and many of the other boys had also eaten the potatoes, without coming to any harm.

The possible causes could be further narrowed down. There had been two sittings for the meal, and all the boys who were taken ill had attended the first sitting. These were the younger pupils, and it appeared that the youngest boys of all, who were served first, were the ones who suffered most. There were no cases among those who attended the second sitting, nor among the boys who ate their meal in a smaller room adjacent to the dining room, nor among teachers or kitchen staff. But one or two of the older boys who monitored the first sitting were also affected.

In the food store-room adjacent to the kitchen were several sacks (50 kg) of potatoes arranged neatly in rows along the wall. These were delivered weekly, and the potatoes in question had arrived only three days before term began. Three quarters of a sack were used each day. In the far corner of the store-room was a single, smaller paper bag full of potatoes, which was still tied up and had apparently never been opened. The kitchen staff said that it, and another sack, had been left over from the end of the summer term. The other sack had been opened and inspected by the chef, but declared unfit for consumption and removed from the store-room for disposal.

The procedure for preparing the potatoes was to carry them in a bucket from the store-room to the peeling machine in the kitchen, and this required four separate bucketfuls. The peeling machine accommodated only one bucketful at a time, and discharged the peeled potatoes into a bowl, where one of the kitchen staff removed eyes and blemishes by hand. While this has was being done, the next bucketful was being peeled in the peeling machine.

The four bowls of peeled potatoes were then tipped into two large pans for boiling. When the potatoes were cooked they were tipped from the pans into five shallow serving dishes—three filled from one pan, and two from the other. The first serving dish, which was set aside for the teachers, was kept warm in the kitchen oven. Potatoes from this dish were also eaten later by the kitchen staff. Since neither of these groups fell ill, this batch was clearly not the culprit. The other four serving dishes were placed in a heated container in the boy's dining room, and removed to a serving counter one by one, as required.

The older boys who supervised the dining hall were served first, and then the youngest boys. Each boy on average received a helping of two potatoes. Then came the boys in the next grade up. At the end of the first sitting, the hall was cleared and the more senior boys and those eating in the side room came in for the second sitting. They all remained well.

The only possible explanation for the illnesses was that, despite what the kitchen staff said, one bucketful of old potatoes had been used that day, and the sack containing these had been opened first. They would have been peeled together, and although they were boiled in the same pan as a bucket of the newer potatoes, it is likely that they sat at the bottom of the pan. They would then have been transferred together into one of the five serving dishes. Only the dinner monitors and the first group of boys who were served from this dish would have been affected.

This theory was proved by scientific analysis on some of the boiled potatoes recovered from the refuse bin two days later. The symptoms were typical of a toxin that affected the body's acetyl cholinesterase, the essential enzyme that facilitates the transmission of nerve impulses from one nerve ending to another. The anti-cholinesterase activity of the extract obtained from the recovered potatoes was examined by a leading specialist, Dr Mary Whittaker of King's College, London, and she found that it inhibited the cholinesterase enzyme three times as strongly as a control extract prepared from fresh potatoes. She estimated that the recovered potatoes contained 25–30 mg of solanine per 100 g of boiled potato—enough to cause the symptoms in the boys who are them. The case was solved.

In an outbreak of poisoning 20 years earlier, reported by Graham Wilson in the *Monthly Bulletin of the Ministry of Health*, four people repeatedly became ill through eating potatoes. In this case they ate the skin as well as the flesh of the baked potatoes, and fell ill about eight hours after their meal. This time interval is short for bacterial food poisoning, and resembles that in the school outbreak. These people's symptoms too were vomiting, abdominal pain, diarrhoea, and malaise. They showed no neurological symptoms and were less severely affected—they recovered each time within 24 hours.

Rarely does solanine kill, but it can happen. In 1918 in Glasgow, Scotland, 61 people were taken ill with headache, vomiting, and diarrhoea a few hours after eating potatoes. One boy, aged five, died the following day of strangulation of the bowel following extreme retching and vomiting. In another outbreak in 1925, seven members of a family were poisoned by greened potatoes, and two of them died. In this case all experienced vomiting and one member of the family suffered from diarrhoea, but none had fever. There was extreme exhaustion, sometimes preceded by restlessness, but no convulsions. Breathing was rapid and laboured, and consciousness was lost a few hours before death.

Massive outbreaks of solanine poisoning occurred in North Korea during the war years of 1952–53, when communities were reduced to eating rotten potatoes. In one area 382 people were affected, of whom 52 entered hospital and 22 died. Those most severely affected died within 24 hours from heart failure. Those slightly less severely affected had weak irregular pulses, enlargement of the heart, pallor of the skin, blueing of lips and ears, and enlargement of the liver. The level of consciousness was normal, but reflexes were slow. Another group also experienced swelling of the face, abdomen, and extremities, and they became inactive and lethargic but not unconscious. Nevertheless, they died within five or ten days. In the final stages there were sometimes a state of high excitability with shaking attacks, and death was due to respiratory failure.

Solanine occurs naturally in potato but usually only in amounts between 3 and 6 mg per 100 g. Most of this is just below the surface, and is removed when the potato is peeled. Amounts of solanine are greatly increased by bruising and by exposure to light that causes greening, and are higher when the potato has begun to sprout. Most people can easily cope with the solanine in the average portion of potatoes, and show no symptoms of poisoning, because the body can break it down and rapidly excrete the products in the urine. But when the level of solanine is high, and it can be as high as 40 mg per 100 g of potato, then we experience a toxic reaction with diarrhoea the main symptom, progressing to difficulty with breathing, and even coma.

The green parts of the potato plant are high in solanine, and yet some groups consume these parts of the plant. For example, people in the UK Bangladeshi community eat potato tops and leaves, and a study of a group of these people showed no toxic effects even though the leaf samples had up to 22 mg of solanine and 55 mg of chaconine per 100 g of potato. This illustrates the human adaptation to diet, and the variable tolerance which occurs in different populations.

But some people are less tolerant of even very low levels of solanine. If you avoid eating potatoes because of the effect they have on you, it may be that you are less able to detoxify solanine than other people. A potato snack, which may consist of only a couple of ounces (50 g) of potato, might be acceptable, but a generous helping of boiled, baked, or fried potatoes could leave you writhing in agony a few hours later.

We have covered food intolerance toward solanine in some detail to show that even the most common of foods may contain a component that our body has to detoxify and remove. But most of us, young and old, can continue to enjoy potatoes, which are a good source of starch, protein, and vitamin C (provided we don't cook them for too long). We should, however, be on the look-out for signs of greening and darkening, and throw away any potatoes that are so affected.

Lectins

Beans are members of the legume family, and they are grown and consumed in vast quantities. Because they are seeds, they are a rich source of all the nutrients that a plant needs to establish itself, which means that they are generally high in protein, carbohydrate, minerals, and an energy reserve in the form of oils. Soya beans are the single most important bean crop: they are grown extensively in China, Japan, and more recently the USA, where a variety has been developed that has a higher fat content—20%—than the traditional variety, which is 7% fat. The global annual production figures for legumes are shown in Table 8.4, and bear out the importance of beans to human nutrition. However, there are hidden dangers in some beans. The non-nutrients they contain can damage the gut wall and other organs, especially if the beans are eaten raw, or when they have young shoots. In 1980 Norman Noah and colleagues at the Communicable Disease Surveillance Centre, London, published a definitive paper in the *British Medical Journal* recounting a number of outbreaks of food poisoning caused by eating uncooked beans.

The first of these cases was in 1976, when a group of schoolboys, aged 17, and three teachers were taken ill on holiday. They had returned to their hostel after a day out, and discovered to their dismay that the chicken which they had intended to eat for their supper was going off. Instead they put together an impromptu meal of salad, hard-boiled eggs, freshly cooked hot potatoes, and raw red kidney beans (*Phaseolus vulgaris*). Normally these beans

Table 8.4 Legume crops.

Crop	Yield (millions of tonnes per annum)
Soya beans	107
Peanuts	23
Dried peas	17
Dried beans	16
Chick peas	6.8
Green peas	4.8
Dried broad beans	4.3
Green beans	3.1
Lentils	2.7

are purchased as dried beans and are left to soak before cooking. In fact, a packet of them had been left under water in a saucepan all day, as the plan had been that they would be cooked and served with the chicken. Instead, a few of the swollen but uncooked beans were now incorporated into the salad. The beans were not popular, and only nine of the group ate them. Between one and one-and-a-half hours later, all nine began to vomit, with diarrhoea developing somewhat later. The two boys with the worst symptoms were admitted to hospital, and one needed an intravenous infusion. Recovery was rapid in all cases, but what had caused this outbreak of food poisoning?

None of the usual food-poisoning bacteria was isolated from the faeces or vomit of the patients, so food poisoning could be ruled out. The speedy onset of the symptoms meant that a virus was not the cause either. An unopened packet of beans was analysed, and a possible culprit, the bacterium *Bacillus cereus*, was identified as present, but the extent of contamination was much too small to have caused the illness. The beans were also analysed for the toxic metals arsenic, mercury, and lead, but only the normal low levels of these were present; the same was true of cyanide. The Mycological Reference Laboratory was sent a sample of the beans and were able to isolate *Trichoderma* and *Penicillium*, but neither of these moulds was thought likely to have caused the outbreak.

At about the same time, other incidents were reported. Again in 1976, nine people were ill with nausea, vomiting, and diarrhoea when they ate white beans that had been soaked in water and eaten raw; two were hospitalised and one was seriously ill. A similar incident occurred in 1979, only this time red beans were involved, and 15 people became ill. The incubation period before the onset of symptoms was 1–3 hours, but recovery was complete and rapid. The smallest 'dose' to produce symptoms was four beans. That same year another case showed that red beans could be poisonous even when they were casseroled in a slow cooker, set at the 'low' setting, for two-and-a-half hours, before a portion was eaten. The remainder was eaten after a further three hour's cooking, but they still caused symptoms.

In all these incidents faecal samples from the patients, and samples of the beans themselves, were examined, but no pathogens were isolated that could account for the symptoms. The cause of all these cases was a group of natural toxins called lectins. Lectins are a group of proteins produced by plants. They are widely distributed in nature, especially in seeds, although their function is not clear. In the human body they cause a variety of responses: some cause clotting of the blood, and others interfere with the immune system leading to inflammation, particularly of the gut wall. Some lectins are carcinogenic.

A sample of beans that had caused vomiting and diarrhoea in one outbreak were examined for lectins, and were shown to contain 19 mg per gram of dry weight, which is enough to cause anyone eating them to become ill. Uncooked beans can contain much higher levels, over 50 mg per gram. When these are soaked in water for several hours, about two-thirds of the lectins are leached out—thus an initial level of 50 mg in the red beans is reduced to less than 20 mg after soaking. Cooking will then remove most of the remaining lectins.

White kidney beans, another variety of *Phaseolus vulgaris*, contain slightly less toxin— namely, 17 mg per gram—but very little of this is lost when they are soaked, and so they end up being just as poisonous if eaten raw. Broad beans (*Vicia faba*) on the other hand, contain much smaller amounts of lectin, only 3 gm per gram, and this remains unchanged even after soaking. At this level our detoxification system can cope easily, and we can enjoy this vegetable with our meals.

If you have ever eaten red or white kidney beans and were sick afterwards, while others eating the same food appeared to be all right, you might have assumed you were allergic to the beans. What is more likely is that you are intolerant of the residual lectins they contained. While your companions coped by virtue of successful detoxification, your metabolism could not muster enough resources to deal with the poison, and so resorted to the more violent expedient of expelling the offending food from the gut.

When raw, unsoaked red or white beans were fed to rats as 80% of their diet, all the animals died within three days. When fed as 40% of the diet then death resulted after 3–11 days, and even when beans comprised only 10% the rats suffered ill effects.

None of the above information should spoil your enjoyment of red or white beans, and indeed they are an enjoyable part of many dishes, such as chilli con carne. If, after soaking, the beans are boiled for 15 minutes, the lectins are destroyed. Beans that are bought ready to use in cans are perfectly safe to eat without further cooking.

Oxalic acid and oxalate

Oxalic acid is the chemical used to remove stains from wooden furniture—it is an essential part of the furniture restorer's trade. It is also much used by boat owners to remove dirt and algae from teak decks, leaving the wood looking like new. Oxalic acid is also a natural toxin, and is found, either as the acid or as derivatives called oxalates, in chocolate, peanuts, spinach, sorrel, parsley, beetroot, and tea.

Too much oxalate causes a sore throat, abdominal pain, diarrhoea, and occasionally vomiting of blood. The kidney becomes damaged and renal failure can follow. Oxalate in the highest concentration occurs in rhubarb leaves (there is less in the stalks) and children are the most commonly poisoned as a result of eating rhubarb leaves. One fatal case of poisoning is known to have occurred as a result of eating sorrel soup. A lesser effect is commonly seen in the spring when an excess of strawberries or rhubarb is eaten: this results in oxalate crystals damaging the kidneys and the ureters, the pipes leading from the kidneys to the bladder. (These crystals may in time develop into kidney stones.) This causes a severe pain in the abdomen which is called renal or ureteric colic. The kidneys can take several weeks to recover, but there is no long-term damage.

The ordinary diet delivers between 80–100 mg of oxalate a day. Most of this is not absorbed by the body, because in the intestines it forms insoluble calcium oxalate and is carried out with the faeces. In the condition known as hyperoxaluria, however, there is oxalate excretion in the urine, showing that this toxin is being absorbed. Increased absorption can occur when the calcium in food is tied up with other dietary components, such as fatty acids, if these are poorly digested due to intestinal disease or as a result of surgery. The best way to avoid oxalate poisoning and kidney stones is to limit fat intake, increase calcium intake, drink more fluids, and restrict the intake of oxalate by avoiding foods that contain significant amounts: beans in tomato sauce, leeks, beetroot, green peppers, spinach, blackberries, gooseberries, red currants, rhubarb, beer, tea, chocolate, and peanuts provide more than 15 mg of oxalate at a typical serving. In terms of milligrams of oxalate per 100 g of food, those foods with the highest amounts are: stewed rhubarb (860), spinach (750), beetroot (675), and cocoa powder (620). Other foods with moderate amounts of oxalate include runner beans, broad beans, celery, and strawberries. Foods with no oxalate are bread, milk, eggs, cheese, most other vegetables and fruits, and cereals.

HCAs and PAHs

As soon as humans began to cook food they improved their diet, and this brought major benefits. Cooking aids digestion by disintegrating animal tissues, breaking up the tightly bound granules of starch in cereals, and detoxifying components of plants that were too poisonous to eat raw, such as certain beans. There are some disadvantages, such as the loss of some vitamins, but by and large cooking is enormously beneficial.

Cooking can bring with it other dangers: contact with smoke, which is known to contain cancerous agents; and overcooking meat (roasting) or charring cereals (toasting), which also produce chemicals that have been shown to be carcinogenic to animals. Cooking certain meats at high temperatures creates chemicals that are not found in raw meat, and some of them may increase the risk of cancer. Attention has come to focus on a group known as the heterocyclic amines (HCAs), which have been found in the overcooked muscle meat of beef, pork, fowl, and fish. So far researchers in Japan have identified 17 different types of HCA, and other researchers in Europe have found HCAs in meats cooked in a variety of ways, the common factor in their production being the high temperature. Thus broiling, barbecuing, and frying meats produce the greatest amounts of HCAs, although this depends very much on the time taken to cook them. A threefold increase in HCAs occurs when the oven temperature is raised from 200 to 250 °C (400 °F to 480 °F). The gravies made from the juices of meats cooked this way also have high levels of HCAs. Stewing, boiling, and poaching of meat produces negligible amounts of HCAs, as does cooking in a microwave oven.

In 1992, the US National Cancer Institute conducted an epidemiological survey of 176 people diagnosed with stomach cancer and analysed their cooking and eating habits. These people were compared with those of 503 controls who had no evidence of cancer. People who liked their beef medium to well done, and who were thereby exposed to high levels of HCAs, had more than three times the incidence of stomach cancer compared to those who ate beef rare or medium-rare. In addition, the incidence was twice as great in those who ate beef four times per week, compared to those ate it less often. Other work showed that the incidence of colorectal, pancreatic, and breast cancer was higher in those who ate lots of well-done, fried, or barbecued meat.

The browning of carbohydrate-rich foods, like sugar and bread, on cooking and baking is not due to the production of charred organic matter, but is the result of chemical reactions that carbohydrates undergo when heated. Consequently there is no formation of HCAs, but there is of PAHs, the polycyclic aromatic hydrocarbons. These form another group of potentially cancerous chemicals, of which around a hundred types have been identified in barbecued and toasted foods. PAHs are not only formed in cooking: they are also formed when anything organic burns, and they are present in asphalt, so they contaminate urban environments, albeit in tiny amounts. And nature also makes them on a worldwide scale in plants and microorganisms on land and in the sea, and they are injected into the atmosphere when volcanoes erupt and forests burn. They form a tiny part of all our diets, and the proportion in food is measured in parts per billion (p.p.b.). They are present at 1 p.p.b. in barbecued beef, grilled steak, smoked fish, and coffee at which level they present no threat; but it is their raised level in charcoal-grilled steak at 8 p.p.b. that has been a cause for concern. Rats fed charcoal-grilled beef, however, showed no more stomach tumours than those fed only on raw beef or soya bean meal, and it seems likely that PAHs are not a reason to change our eating habits.

CHAPTER 9

Additives and contaminants

Many farmed and processed foods contain small amounts of substances that have been added, either intentionally or unintentionally, during production. They contribute little to the nutritional value of the food, but may nevertheless have an effect on some of the people who eat them. These unnatural non-nutrients fall into two main categories: additives and contaminants.

Additives are chemicals that are purposely put into food to enhance its appearance, acceptability, palatability, and quality. Some might disagree with the last attribute, believing all food additives to be contaminants. This may have once been the case, when food adulteration was commonplace; and even today, contaminants may be present. However, these are defined as chemicals that have polluted food by accident, as a result of agricultural methods or factory processing.

Food additives

Some additives, such as flavour, flavour-enhancers, sweeteners, and colouring agents, are put into foods merely for cosmetic purposes. Some are there to stop food going rancid, such as the antioxidants added to edible oils, and some are there to prevent emulsions, like mayonnaise, from separating back into oil and vinegar. Some are there to prevent powders from caking, and to keep them free-flowing. Some additives control the acidity of a product, some produce the smooth texture we expect of ice-cream, and some are needed if the product is to be sold as a gel. Some additives are more like ingredients, and have been used for hundreds of years, such as raising agents in flour. Quite unexpected chemicals are to be found in lists of approved additives. For example, vitamin C (listed as ascorbic acid) is used in bread-making to improve the texture of the dough. Sadly, none of this survives into the final loaf.

The modification of some foods today starts even before the sowing of the seed, with genetic engineering and the culture of pest-resistant species. From that point onwards humans interfere with nature at every step, right up to the time the food is on the end of a fork. This is not necessarily a bad thing, although some would have us believe otherwise. The most troublesome of all food additives is sulfur dioxide, which has been dealt with in Chapter 8, but even that is only a hazard for susceptible people, or when it is present in unusually high quantities. The same is true of most additives. Generally the benefits far out-weigh the risks: additives enable food to be transported thousands of miles yet still arrive fresh; and flavour, colour, and consistency can all be improved using the additives involved in modern food processing techniques. The amounts of synthetic materials added are a small proportion of the intake of non-nutrients that the body has to cope with, and all these additives have been fully tested and shown to be harmless. The US Food and Drug Administration (FDA) classifies them as 'generally regarded as safe', or GRAS for short; and chemicals which do not come into this category often have strict limits imposed on their use.

As well as the FDA, there are other organisations that have been active in the area of food additives. For example, the UK has its Food Advisory Committee of the Ministry of Agriculture, Fisheries, and Food (MAFF), and the European Union (EU) has a Community Regulations and Directives Directorate. Since 1986, all processed foods in the EU must carry a list of additives in addition to the ingredients—the additives are listed either by their chemical name, or by a so-called E-number. Lists of E-numbers are published officially, but they are also to be found in books such as *Understanding Additives* published by the UK Consumer's Association (Hodder and Stoughton, 1988). Table 9.1 shows the broad cate-gories of additives, and their designated codes. The American Dietetic Association's *Complete Food & Nutrition Guide* also has useful information about food additives, although these are not E-number coded as in Europe.

The World Health Organisation also takes an active interest in additives. Its Worldwide Codex Alimentarius Commission, which has 123 member countries, has four main aims: to protect the health of consumers and ensure fair practice in the food trade; to promote inter-national standards and coordinate these between member countries; to set priorities and prepare draft standards; and to finalise agreed standards and publish them in the *Codex*

Table 9.1 Categories of food additives and their code numbers.

The European number	Category
E100–E180	colours
E200–E290	preservatives
E300–E322	anti-oxidants
E400–E483*	emulsifiers and stabilisers
E905–E907	mineral hydrocarbons
E1400–E1442	modified starches
*E420–E421	sweeteners

Alimentarius. However, there is little chance now that anything harmful, or indeed any new additive, will ever be added to the lists of permitted additives because the cost of testing is prohibitive, including as it does several types of laboratory animal. Unless a new additive were to offer something exceptionally beneficial, it is unlikely that it would justify the cost of testing.

Case study: **Happy birthday blues**

Sarah's mother had noticed a change in her daughter's behaviour over a period of twelve months. Sarah had been particularly irritable at her tenth birthday party, when she came to blows with one of her friends. This was most uncharacteristic of her. Her brother and sister, both older, had never misbehaved so badly. The family were all musical, and Sarah was learning the violin. Until recently she had enjoyed playing and practising with the family but now she found it difficult to concentrate or sit still. Even at play she was clearly disturbed, and was unable to do anything for any length of time. Sarah's parents decided to consult a behaviour therapist.

On questioning the parents, it appeared there were no family problems, and while Sarah's school work had deteriorated, there was no evidence of bullying. When the questioning turned to her diet, her parents' answers soon revealed the likely cause of the change in behaviour. Sarah had become more adventurous in her eating habits, but not in a healthy direction. Her basic diet was nutritionally sound and diverse, but she was allowed to indulge in a variety of savoury snacks, flavoured crisps (potato chips), orange and blackcurrant fruit drinks, fruit yoghurts, and chewy fruit-flavoured sweets. It seemed likely that this overload of high-additive foods was at the root of Sarah's problems.

Consequently Sarah was placed on an 'additive-free' diet, and despite the loss of most of her daily treats, she co-operated and agreed to substitute fresh fruit, plain crisps, and fresh fruit juices. Six weeks later her mother reported that she was back to her old self: even an hour-long session of violin practice was not a problem, and there had been no more temper tantrums. The implication was that an excess of non-nutrient additives had been the cause of Sarah's hyperactivity.

The most common and probably the most contentious additives are those that are connected to hyperactivity or attention deficit syndrome in young children, of the kind illustrated in the box. The hyperactive child comes in all shades. At one extreme there are severely handicapped children, while at the other are those with a variety of behavioural problems. The typical hyperactive child may be constantly on the move or fidgeting, and they may touch or handle everything, or everybody, around them and then quickly move on to something else. Some of them rock back and forth or have other repetitive movements, and they will not sleep easily, often pounding their pillows. Mood swings are common, with panics or temper tantrums, and they become easily frustrated. This leads inevitably to failure in what they are trying to do, causing further frustration. Sometimes they are clumsy, running into things, and breaking their toys. Lastly, their attention span may be so short as to make learning difficult, and yet when tested their IQ may be above average or even quite high.

What causes a child to become hyperactive? Some say it is due to poor parenting, and others look for psychological explanations, while some believe that the answer lies in the child's diet. Those who target food as the root of the problem can point to the dramatic results that can follow as a result of choosing the right diet. Whether this improvement is real can be tested, by reintroducing some of the suspected items in the diet and noting whether the child's behaviour changes. The results can be spectacular.

Possible links between behaviour and diet were first mooted in the early 1960s by Ben Feingold, an allergist in San Francisco, and Robert Makarness, an English allergist and author of *Not all in the Mind*. The hyperactive children who were accepted for treatment under the new type of regime proposed by Richard Makarness, were placed on elimination diets,* and they showed a marked improvement. However, the results were criticised on the grounds that the method lacked scientific rigour. It was argued that, as with drug development, there should be controlled trials and randomisation of treatment. In other words, the parents and children should not know whether suspect chemicals had been eliminated from the diet.

In response, Feingold and Makanress argued that this relegated the skilled judgement of experienced clinicians to an inferior role. There were other people in the drug world who disliked the 'scientific approach' to the subject: for instance, in 1966 Sir Austin Bradford-Hill, an early advocate of controlled clinical trials who was responsible for the first such trial in the UK said: 'Given the right attitude of mind, there is more than one way we can study therapeutic efficacy. Any belief that the controlled trial is the only way, would mean not that the pendulum had swung too far, but that it had come right off its hook.'

However, the controlled trial remains the corner-stone of the judgement of efficacy, so controlled trials soon followed. Though they were far less conclusive, many of the trials demonstrated some beneficial effect of diet modification.

Children were tested by age and level of exposure, and there appeared to be an association between a diet free of colouring agents and a decrease in hyperactive symptoms. The efficacy levels varied from 30 to 90%, which would fit with the crude designs that are necessary when testing food and its constituents. The additives that were fingered as guilty were few in number, but they were consistently found to be implicated.

In 1985, Joe Egger and colleagues in Professor John Soothill's department at Great Ormond Street Hospital For Sick Children, in London, conducted a controlled trial with all kinds of food challenges, not just additives, and showed a clear association between hyperactive behaviour and food. A food challenge usually follows an elimination diet: an offending agent is reintroduced under clinical supervision. The children were carefully classified and rated for their hyperactivity using a well-recognised scale called the Connor's rating scale. Top of Egger's list of offending agents were the colourants and preservatives, with a

---

*An elimination diet is a regime in which specific elements are removed while keeping the remainder of the diet unchanged.

79% positive correlation between the Connor rating and these kinds of additives, followed by soya, milk, chocolate, grapes, and wheat. The two most common additives that were implicated were the orange dye tartrazine, and the preservative, benzoic acid.

In Australia, Anne Swain and Robert Loblay pursued a similar line of investigation, and discovered that a range of chemicals could produce reactions in susceptible children. The usual pattern was sensitivity to four or five chemicals, but these varied with the child. Swain believed that there was a threshold level that had to be breached before these chemicals caused hyperactivity, and this would fit with the hypothesis that the level of the detoxifying enzyme, cytochrome P450, varies from individual to individual. If there comes a point at which this enzyme can no longer cope, the threshold is exceeded and the child becomes hyperactive.

Another project on children with hyperactivity symptoms was conducted by James Swanson at the Hospital for Sick Children, Toronto, where he and his colleagues examined the effect of *combinations* of colouring agents. On two days of the experiment the children were given a mixture of three colouring agents, and learning tests on those days showed poorer results compared to days on which the children were given a placebo. This work also supports the idea of there being a threshold for detoxification, which may well account for the day-to-day variations in hyperactive children. Accumulation of additives awaiting detoxification would occur, maybe over several days, before a reaction is seen, although it may be possible to trigger a response with one large dose. This failure to detoxify a non-nutrient is not an allergy response, and improvement will come simply by lowering the intake to below that child's threshold. Individuals vary, and for some children the threshold may be very low. But only a relatively few, very susceptible, children are at risk. Before seeking the answer to a child's unacceptable behaviour in his or her diet, parents should first consider the more likely stresses that their child is reacting to, such as marriage breakdown, poor disciplining, lack of constructive play with other children, or bullying at school. If these can be ruled out, then diet may be the reason.

So which are the additives that have been shown to cause a reaction?

Tartrazine (E102)

Tartrazine is one of a class of dyes known as the azo dyes, which were discovered in Germany in the nineteenth century and were found to be ideal for dyeing wool and silk. Azo dyes get their name—and their intensely bright colours—from a nitrogen-to-nitrgoen double bond at the heart of the molecule. Because their colours are so intense, little is needed to achieve the desired degree of coloration. Earlier this century tartrazine began to be used in orange-flavoured drinks because its colour closely resembled the natural colour of oranges, and once it had FDA approval as a food additive it became widely used in a variety of foods. It has been used in bread crumbs, canned vegetables, fish fingers, fish cakes, smoked fish, cakes, biscuits (cookies), sweets, mixed peel, marzipan, ice cream, custard powder, artificial cream, coffee whitener, packet soups, jellies (gelatin desserts), gravy granules, fruit sauces, milk shakes, and soft drinks. Tartrazine is still used in some foods, beverages, cosmetics, and medicines, though to a much lesser degree. Tartrazine-like compounds occur naturally in some foods.

Adverse reactions to tartrazine are more common in people who also react badly to salicylate (see Chapter 6). This dual sensitivity does not always occur, but it is probably due to the fact that tartrazine and salicylate are detoxified by the same elimination pathway. The worst reaction to tartrazine that has been reported was anaphylactic shock, and it happened in a patient who was known to be allergic to tartrazine. It came about as a result of eating jelly beans in combination with medicines and cheese containing the yellow dye. This is an example of chemical triggers, where allergic patients suffer unduly because of the susceptibility of their cells to non-specific, non-allergic triggering mechanisms. More likely reactions to tartrazine involve swelling of the face, lips, and throat (angio-oedema), urticaria asthma, and rhinitis.

How likely is a child to be sensitive to tartrazine? The answer is: very unlikely. It is estimated that only one child in ten thousand will be affected, which is less likely than being born as one of triplets. Nevertheless the risk is there, and this colorant has been withdrawn in the USA because it is a recognised sensitizer. Although it is still a permitted additive in the UK, very little is actually used.

Erythrosine (E127)

Erythrosine is a red dye used in cherries, gelatines, ice cream, fruit cocktails, sherbet, cereals, chocolate, garlic sausage, and salamis. It belongs to the family of chemicals called xanthenes, and is water-soluble. The average intake is about 8 mg per day, of which about 20% is absorbed. However, erythrosine is excreted in the bile and therefore back into the gut, so it can be absorbed again. Animal experiments have shown it to interfere with the central nervous system, and other research has demonstrated fine changes in the function of the thyroid glands because of it. This might explain how it can modify behaviour, but no definitive mechanism for such interference has been identified. Nevertheless, challenge studies with erythrosine have shown it to cause hyperactive behaviour in susceptible children.

Cochineal (E120)

Cochineal is a natural red dye derived from cactus beetles, and is the colorant used in some traditional foods such as garlic sausage. It is also used in some alcoholic drinks. Excess cochineal intake has also been linked to hyperactivity in children, as has a synthetic version, Ponceau 4R (E124) which is known as cochineal red A. Although this is the same colour as cochineal, and was given this name because of it, there is no chemical similarity between the two. Ponceau 4R is an ingredient in packet soups, seafood dressings, desert toppings, salami, and quick-setting jellies/gelatins. It should be avoided by people who are sensitive to aspirin, and those who are asthmatic.

Other chemical colouring agents Other chemical colouring agents that have occasionally been suspected of causing adverse reactions leading to hyperactivity are: allura red, amaranth (E123), brilliant black (E151), brilliant blue (E133), brilliant scarlet (E124), carmosine (E122), chocolate brown (E155), green S (E142), indigo carmine (E132), patent blue (E131), quinoline yellow (E104), sunset yellow (E110), and yellow 2G (E107).

Benzoic acid and benzoates (E210–E219)

Preservatives are another group of chemicals added to food, and many of these are derived from the natural preservatives found in soft fruits such as gooseberries, raspberries, strawberries, and blackcurrants. In these fruits the main natural preservatives are the benzoates. Those most used as food additives are sodium benzoate (E211) and the ethyl and methyl esters of *para*-hydroxybenzoate (E214 and E218), known collectively as parabens. Because benzoates are found naturally and work so well, synthetic variants were introduced, both as flavouring agents and as preservatives. The vast majority of cosmetics also contain parabens as preservatives, especially methyl and propyl parabenzoates (E216).

Thousands of tons of benzoic acid and benzoates are produced each year, and benzoic acid is one of the commonest preservatives in use today. The acid is the active form, and benzoate salts will convert to benzoic acid in the acidic conditions of the stomach. Benzoic acid is rapidly absorbed by the body and detoxified in the liver, ending up as the metabolite hippuric acid, which then exits in the urine. There is an average daily outflow of 0.7 g.

Benzoic acid prevents bacterial and fungal spoilage, and it has been a part of the food industry for almost a century. Quite high levels of benzoic acid can be present naturally, because the processing and concentrating of many foods greatly increases the proportion. This is what happens, for example, when tomatoes are turned into tomato ketchup. Whereas fresh tomatoes may not cause hyperactivity in children, or headaches in adults, the more concentrated forms, such as ketchups, soups, or purées, can produce these effects, and challenge tests have revealed that too much benzoic acid may be a contributing factor.

Because benzoic acid and benzoates are so widely used, it is not surprising that a few individuals experience problems with them. But this fact went unrecognised for decades. A hundred years ago benzoates were used for the treatment of rheumatic disorders, and doses of up to 60 g (2 ounces) per day were prescribed, apparently without ill effects. In 1933 a test for liver function in thyroid disease, pregnancy, and other conditions involved the intravenous use of 6 g of sodium benzoate, again with few adverse reactions. Then in 1944 the first anaphylaxis-like response was reported, and this followed the ingestion of a dose given orally. Within a few hours the patient was suffering severe breathlessness, chest pain, and high blood pressure, followed by coma and shock. The patient recovered after two days, and surprisingly the physicians repeated the test, only to find the patient suffered exactly the same symptoms. If they were to do this today, they would almost certainly be accused of malpractice, and sued.

The ensuing years saw more and more reports of adverse reactions to benzoic acid and benzoates, and many studies have been conducted under stringent scientific control. These have demonstrated the various symptoms that susceptible people exhibit. According to Alexander Fisher and Lea Febiger's *Contact Dermatitis*, benzoates cause reactions in the skin with urticaria and angio-oedema. There is evidence from a wide range of studies that cross-over reactivity can occur: patients with salicylate sensitivity react to benzoates.

When benzoates come into contact with the skin of people who are sensitive to it, there is immediate wealing and flaring. This suggests an allergic or immune response, with symptoms caused by the release of histamine. However, it is not an allergic or immune response, because on repeated applications of benzoic acid the effect wears off. If the skin is then scratched with histamine it will still react, suggesting that wealing is caused by the release of another reactive substance (probably serotonin), which becomes depleted with repeated applications. Also, in susceptible people, the reactions in the skin were not blocked by prior dosing with antihistamine drugs.

Another symptom which is confined almost exclusively to patients who suffer from asthma, is increased breathlessness and wheezing when challenged with benzoates. In 1977, 272 asthmatic patients were tested and eleven of these reported adverse effects. Other studies have produced similar results: around 4% of asthmatics appear to be sensitive to benzoates, which means that for the population as a whole this is likely to be a rare condition. Few people are affected, which is fortunate given the wide use of benzoates in food, beverages, drugs, and cosmetics.

Sorbic acid and sorbates (E200—E203)

Sorbic acid and sorbates are naturally occurring chemicals that occur in some berries, such as those of the tree *Sorbis americana*, which is commonly known as mountain ash. Sorbic acid is an effective antimicrobial agent, and is used as a food preservative at levels of 0.1–0.3% (at which it is odourless and tasteless). It is particularly effective against yeasts and moulds, and is to be found in a wide range of foods, including jellies (gelatin desserts), wines, dried fruits, and cheese and cheese products. In some people it causes skin problems such as rashes, angio-oedema, and a non-allergic urticaria that is not blocked by antihistamines. Sorbic acid has also been shown to produce an allergic eczema: this was first reported in a baker, and was traced to the flour he used, which contained sorbic acid that had been added as a preservative. Excessive amounts of sorbates will produce a stinging around the mouth, which is caused by the release of a chemical that affects blood vessels. People susceptible to sorbic acid experience these effects with much lower degrees of exposure.

Antioxidants (E300—E321)

Oxidation can affect the flavour of foods containing fat, which slowly becomes rancid as it reacts with the oxygen in the atmosphere. Antioxidants are preservatives which delay the onset of rancidity, so that edible oils, and foods derived from them, remain untainted for weeks and months. Some antioxidants are not only natural, but also beneficial in their own right: the commonly used antioxidant ascorbic acid (E300) is better known as vitamin C.

When ascorbic acid is used in this way it is added as a fat-soluble derivative called ascorbyl palmitate. An alternative is vitamin E (α-tocopherol) which, despite its higher cost, is also becoming popular. This is naturally present in many vegetable oils. Other oils have their own natural antioxidants, such as avenasterol in olive oil, and others, as yet unidentified, in sesame seed oil. Research to identify these could lead to their widespread use as well. It is thought that these natural antioxidants might protect against cancer.

Different foods require different antioxidants. Those used for fats and oils must be fat-soluble, and the two most commonly used today are butylated hydroxyanisole, BHA (E320), and butylated hydroxytoluene, BHT (E321). They are added up to a level of 200 p.p.m., which is 0.02%. They are not permitted in foods intended for babies, except in certain cases where the fat-soluble vitamin A needs to be protected. Adverse reactions are extremely rare, but BHA and BHT have caused eczema and non-specific rashes in susceptible people. Other symptoms are rhinitis, wheezing, headache, sleepiness, chest pain, flushing, and red eyes. BHA and BHT have been shown to have anti-cancer properties, at least in laboratory animals, and would probably act to protect humans as well. They are thought to work by stimulating the enzymes that destroy free radicals (see the Glossary).

The usefulness of antioxidants is their ability to preserve food that would otherwise go rancid, and this consideration far outweighs the occasional problems they cause to a few luckless individuals.

The gallates (E310–E312)

Gallates are used as preservatives in breakfast cereals, snack foods, and chewing gum, and they can affect asthma sufferers, mainly causing painful dyspepsia. Octyl gallate is used to preserve fats, oils, and margarine. It can cause gastric irritation, and is not allowed in foods for babies.

The other main class of additives is the emulsifiers, and the most common example is the polysorbs.

Polysorbs (E432–436)

The five polysorb compounds, which are made from the ethylene oxide and sorbitan esters, are widely used in cakes as emulsifiers and stabilisers. They have all been rigorously tested and are used in many kinds of foods. Polysorbs are found in sweets, ice creams, coffee whiteners, artificial creams, and toppings. The incidence of problems with them is so rare that any risk is far outweighed by their usefulness.

Table 9.2 lists the few other additives where adverse reactions have been reported. By now you might be wondering whether greater checks should be made on the safety of food additives. It is our contention that the majority of these chemicals are perfectly safe, and the incidence of problems associated with a small number of them are as low as, if not lower

Table 9.2 Other food additives which can cause adverse effects.

Additive	Code number	Adverse reaction
Agar	E404	abdominal distension or obstruction
Ammonium persulfate	n.a.	Baker's eczema
Calcium disodium EDTA	E385	vomiting, diarrhoea, abdominal pain
Carrageenan	E407	implicated in ulcerative colitis
Glycerol	E422	headache, thirst, nausea
Mannitol	E421	nausea, vomiting, diarrhoea
Potassium chloride	E508	gut ulceration, haemorrhage, perforation
Propylene glycol	n.a.	flare up of dermatitis
Tragacanth	E413	contact dermatitis

than, those associated with naturally occurring non-nutrients. In fact, the natural varieties are consumed in far greater quantities, and have much more power to affect us—as the previous chapter demonstrated.

Any non-nutrient chemical in excess is potentially hazardous, but the same is true of many nutrients. The body has a very efficient system for dealing with non-nutrients, and only if our metabolism is compromised in some way will an overdose pose a threat. Considering the extensive testing that the food industry undertakes, and the stringent regulations in force, we are better protected today than ever before. Indeed, we would be far worse off if food were not modified by these additives. Colouring agents have a psychological impact but they are nevertheless important in making food look attractive to eat.

Nitrates and nitrites

Nitrates and nitrites are additives commonly used in food processing, and so are not contaminants themselves; however, in some foods during cooking they can be converted into nitrosamines, contaminants that are suspected of causing cancer.

Nitrate consists of a nitrogen atom surrounded by three oxygen atoms, and nitrite has two oxygen atoms. Enzymes convert nitrate to nitrite as part of the nitrogen cycle in the environment, and in living things. Both compounds have been used for many years to cure hams, bacon, and corned beef to protect them against bacteria, and, in the case of boiled ham and sausages, they also give the product an attractive pink hue. The levels of nitrates and nitrites are strictly controlled—nitrite to 200 p.p.m. and nitrate to 500 p.p.m.—but they are needed because they are highly effective in killing the bacteria that cause botulinum poisoning. Although heating would kill *Clostridium botulinum*, the heat would have to penetrate to the spores deep within the meat, and this would spoil the outer layers by overcooking. Instead, nitrite does the job.

Food contaminants

Some components in food get there by accident, and are known as contaminants. They may or may not represent dangers, but we have yet to discover their long-term effects, if any. We know what the contaminants are, we know where they are coming from, and we may even have a very good idea where they end up, but whether they might do us harm is unknown, although clearly they represent no short-term threat.

Speculation about contaminants has fuelled many food scares in the past, and we are right to remain on alert until science or time proves them safe. Studies on animals exposed to huge doses or to small doses over long periods reassure us that the contaminants tested are safe, but this research cannot provide information about what minute doses do to human beings over a lifetime. We may use epidemiological studies as a guideline, but the results of these surveys may be little better than inspired guess work.

Metal contaminants

The harmful metals most likely to contaminte food are lead, mercury, and cadmium. Until recently aluminium would also have been on this list: high levels had been detected in the brains of people who died of Alzheimer's disease, and for many years aluminium was assumed to be a cause of the disease. Books were written warning people of the dangers of the metal, and people campaigned to have it excluded from any process that involved food or drinking water. Then came the discovery that the early analyses for aluminium had grossly exaggerated the amount that was present. Everyone had been misled, and a complex theory of cause and effect had been constructed on faulty data, with the result that for 20 years food writers and broadcasters had been giving out meaningless advice about the dangers of aluminium. Today it is no longer regarded as a health hazard.

   Such a reprieve is never going to happen for lead, mercury, and cadmium: the evidence for their toxicity is too well founded. Lead has been used extensively for centuries, and particularly in this century, when it has been widely used to boost fuel efficiency as an anti-knock agent in gasoline. This use is now being phased out, and will join the many other historical uses of lead that were once common but which threaten us no longer, such as pewter tableware, water pipes, paints, and ceramics. In all cases it has been possible to find much safer alternatives, such as copper and plastics for pipes. Yet accidental poisoning can occur and lead can get into our food in expected, if uncommon ways. Game birds can contain lead shot; moonshine spirits are sometimes made using an old lead-soldered car radiator as a still; and pottery glaze that has been under-fired can release lead, as the case study in the box shows.

Case study: **Cool, refreshing—and deadly**

Michael is a successful businessman living and working in Madrid, where he and his wife Liz have an apartment in an old block dating back to the sixteenth century. When he was in his mid-thirties, and enjoying the good life, Michael noticed that he was losing weight, although this was not intentional. The weight loss was slow at first, but then over a period of months it accelerated until he had lost almost 25 kg (around 50 lb). This loss had been accompanied by a change in bowel habits: he had become increasingly constipated, and often suffered severe cramping abdominal pain.

   One day Michael rang his brother, a doctor living in England, and described his symptoms, and he was immediately told to return to the UK. His brother met him, saw how ill he looked, and straight away drove him to the nearest large hospital. Blood tests revealed the highest levels of lead the hospital had experienced, and when Liz returned to the UK it was was found that she too had toxic levels of lead, but only one fifth as high as her husband's.

   Michael was treated to remove the lead from his system, and advised to examine his environment when he returned home. Back in Madrid he first went to the Public Health Department. He was certain that, because his apartment was in an ancient building, it probably had lead pipes, and these would be the cause of his poisoning. However, the official he spoke to had other ideas: 'Señor, you have a cottage in the mountains?' Michael replied that he had. 'Then look to your pottery there,' was the advice.

   For their weekend retreat, Michael and Liz had bought local pottery. One favourite piece was a three-litre jug which fitted neatly in their fridge, and in which they stored their favourite drink: *sangría*. This was left to chill, and would keep for days. What Michael and Liz had not been aware of was that this jug had a lead glaze that had not been properly fired. One consequence was that the lead leached out and into the *sangría*. The different degrees of poisoning that Michael and Liz experienced reflected the amounts they drank from the fridge, with Liz taking only about one fifth of the amount Michael consumed.

Lead is toxic, but our defences against it are moderately good. It is not easily absorbed across the gut wall, so most of the lead we take in is excreted in our faeces. The lead that is absorbed into the bloodstream is passed through the liver, enters the bile, and goes back into the gut. Nevertheless, a little gets deposited in our bones and teeth, and where it is locked away for a long time, and is almost impossible to eliminate. Our gut is more likely to absorb lead if our diet is low in iron and calcium.

Mercury was a poison commonly found in milliners, since it was used in the treatment of rabbit fur for the production of felt for hats. This explains the old phrase 'mad as a hatter', a condition immortalised by the Victorian author, Lewis Carroll, in the Mad Hatter's Tea Party in *Alice in Wonderland*.

The symptoms of mercury poisoning are shaking, gum bleeding, excessive salivation, and neurological breakdown, and sometimes death. Because the metal has a predilection for brain tissue, mental retardation and developmental defects have also been noted. The organic compounds that mercury forms in nature are difficult to eliminate from the central nervous system, and they can cause permanent neurological damage. The tragedy is not only medical in the acute phase: its victims remain chronically sick, and need support from their families and from society.

The most severe outbreak of mercury poisoning occurred in Japan in the mid-1950s, when a chemical works disposed of its mercury-contaminated effluent in the local bay. No-one realised that it would be converted by microbes to the deadliest form of the metal, methyl mercury, and thereby enter the food chain. Methyl mercury is an organo-mercury compound in which the mercury is directly bonded to a methyl (CH_3) group, which makes it slightly volatile, more mobile, and soluble in fatty tissue. Fish from the bay that were contaminated with methyl mercury provided the locals with much of their protein, and consequently hundreds of people were affected. One of the more distressing symptoms was brain damage caused by the methyl mercury's ability to cross the blood/brain barrier. This particular form of mercury poisoning was called Minamata disease, after the bay, and it killed 143 people.

Other countries, such as Sweden, Pakistan, and Guatemala, have had similar outbreaks of mercury poisoning, due sometimes to accidental contamination, and sometimes to people eating seed grain treated with agrochemical mercury compounds applied to protect it against disease. Mercury poisoning is now almost unheard of in developed societies, but it can still afflict those in developing countries.

Cadmium is also toxic, and there are worries that this metal has so contaminated the environment that it is now a part of everyone's diet. In certain regions around old zinc mines and refineries, the level of cadmium in the soil is so high that local people are warned not to grow and eat their own vegetables. All zinc minerals contain a certain amount of cadmium, and this source of pollution was put into the environment at a time when waste disposal from smelters was not regulated. The use of Moroccan phosphate in fertilizers added to the problem in Europe, because this mineral contained significant amounts of cadmium.

Cadmium was once commonly used to make a bright red pigment (cadmium sulfide) for colouring plastics, and to galvanise iron in place of zinc galvanising because it was much more durable. Even zinc galvanising introduced some cadmium into the environment because the zinc used for this purpose contained a little cadmium. This meant that when galvanized equipment was used in the food industry, some cadmium contamination occurred (now only stainless steel or plastics is allowed in food preparation areas). Today few uses of cadmium are permitted, although it is still a part of long-life batteries; and the WHO has set 0.06 mg per day as a safe limit. The majority of people poisoned by cadmium are those who are exposed to it in the workplace, such as in power stations, battery factories, and the nuclear industry.

While cadmium can be easily absorbed by the body, most ends up in the liver where there are proteins that bind it strongly. The liver's capacity to do this is large, and although we all contain a certain amount of cadmium—the average is about 50 mg—this amount is not life-threatening, nor even a minor health risk.

Nitrosamine contaminants

At one time it was suggested that nitrate was a serious health hazard ('cancer on tap' according to some environmentalists). This alarm came at a time when there were high levels of nitrates in the environment because farmers were applying too much nitrate fertilisers to the land, and it leached into drinking water. Tight controls on the use of such fertilizers now means that little nitrate is lost this way. Some crops, such as lettuce and spinach, absorb and store nitrate, and in this way it gets into the food chain. The human gut itself also produces nitrate, and on a scale which matches that taken in from food and water.

However, nitrates and nitrites can be converted during cooking to the chemically reactive nitrosamines, which animal tests show to be powerful carcinogens. Over the years, nitrosamines have been found in much of our food and drink and some foods are more likely to be contaminated, especially those containing nitrite as a preservative. The smoking of food produces nitrosamines, because it brings together nitrate and amines in warm conditions—a survey in Hong Kong showed nitrosamine levels to be unusually high in smoked fish, salamis, hams, sausage, and bacon. Nitrosamines are also formed, for example, when bacon is fried, although the amounts are tiny.

In larger doses, nitrosamines damage the liver, and this was seen in a man who suffered acute liver damage after industrial exposure to dimethylnitrosamine (DMN). There was an epidemic of liver disease in sheep in the 1960s in Norway, which was traced to the fish meal on which they were fed, and which was laced with the preservative potassium nitrite. This had interacted with the natural fish amines to produce levels of DMN between 30 and 100 p.p.m.

This observation triggered a lot of research into the possibility of human food preserved by nitrite producing high levels of DMN, and so constituting a long-term danger. Proving this is difficult, because it is hard to measure minute levels of nitrosamines accurately; and long-term epidemological data is lacking that might link DMN to diseases like cancer. It is only when nitrate interacts with other food components in animals and fish tissues that nitrosation occurs and the level of DMN rises. DMN has been detected in the stomachs of animals fed only its precursors, and it is therefore a possibility that DMN could also be produced in humans. But it would require a strange set of circumstances for the precursors to come together, namely the right enzymes, the conversion of nitrate to nitrite, and the presence of so-called tertiary amines, so that DMN could form.

Overall, then, it seems that the risk of cancer from the tiny amounts of nitrosamines in our food is very small. However, there is one area of the world where a link between nitrosamines and human cancer is more than tentative: the Transkei region of South Africa, where there is a very high incidence of cancer of the gullet. The area has poor plant production because the soil is deficient in a trace element, molybdenum; and botanists have shown that, without molybdenum, plants accumulate nitrate—the enzyme that maintains an optimal level of plant nitrate has to contain molybdenum, and without the enzyme, the nitrate builds up. This nitrate gets into the human food chain via *Solanum incauum*, a plant that is used extensively to curdle milk. DMN levels in this plant are high. It has been calculated that a ten-year period could provide an intake of 4 mg into the body, far in excess of what would normally be acceptable. Again, this is not *proof* that nitrosamine is responsible for the increased cancers in this region, but it is nevertheless quite compelling evidence, and deserves further investigation.

If there is a risk of cancer from nitrosamines, there is a simple way of reducing it: ensure that your diet includes the antioxidant vitamins A, C, and E, which can destroy nitrosamines. In the USA, the FDA has advised food manufacturers to add these vitamins wherever there is a risk of carcinogens being produced.

Organochlorines

Organochlorine compounds are widely used in industry and agriculture, and so it is not surprising that some of them, such as PCBs and DDT, have found their way into our food. Some people suspect that even exposure to tiny amounts can cause disease in the long term. There is as yet little evidence of this.

PCBs (polychlorinated biphenyls) The PCBs are industrial compounds that were once widely used in engineering as cutting and grinding oils, in electricity transformers as insulating oils, in printing as oils for inks, and in many other processes. They were known to cause an unpleasant skin condition called chloracne, in which the face and hands become covered in pustules, and which was regarded as an industrial disease. But chloracne could be prevented by protective clothing and careful attention to personal hygiene, and meanwhile little care was exercised in the disposal of waste PCBs. As a result, because of their slight volatility, PCBs can now be detected in virtually all parts of the environment and in organisms: they are found in air, water, sediments, fish, land animals, and human tissue—particularly fat and serum.

In 1998, each general practitioner in the UK received a circular from the Chief Medical Officer informing them that PCBs had been found in human breast milk, but that there was no evidence that they constituted any danger. In fact, the presence of PCBs in breast milk has been known for many years, and in the 1980s a joint UN/WHO project compared the PCBs in milk in different countries. High levels were found in Sweden and Germany, and low levels in China, India, and Mexico.

Although detectable amounts of PCBs are present in food, these are so tiny that they are unlikely to provoke an allergic response, or food intolerance. However, larger amounts are toxic. The worst case of PCB poisoning occurred in Japan on the island of Kyushu in 1968, when over 1000 people were affected. The condition became known as Yusho disease (named after the place where it occurred). The cause was contaminated cooking oil, and symptoms included darkened skin, discharging eyes, and chloracne. Babies born to mothers suffering from Yusho disease also showed symptoms. Over 2000 p.p.m. (0.2%) of PCB were found in the cooking oil, and those who consumed the oil still had detectable levels of PCBs in their blood eleven years later.

Recent studies have implicated PCBs in developmental abnormalities in infants whose mothers were exposed to these chemicals during pregnancy. This has also been demonstrated in certain wildlife species. PCBs appear either to be oestrogen-like in the actions they produce in the body, or to affect the hormonal systems indirectly. A large number of toxicological experiments on animals have been carried out using levels of PCBs comparable to the trace levels found in human tissue, but the effects are unclear: sometimes the PCBs behave like an oestrogen, but at other times they act as oestrogen antagonists. There is some evidence of acute poisoning; but there is very little information on the consequences of long-term exposure.

DDT (dichlorodiphenyltrichloroethane)
Today DDT is the most reviled of environmental contaminants, yet it has not always been thought of as insidious poison. Indeed, when it was widely used as a broad-spectrum insecticide, it may well have killed no-one while clearly saving lives by wiping out insects that spread diseases. In the 1940s it was seen as a triumph of scientific endeavour, and the British Prime Minister Winston Churchill described it in one of his famous radio broadcasts as 'an excellent powder...which yields astonishing results.' He was referring to its ability to kill mosquitoes and so prevent malaria in tropical climates. In fact, DDT was found to kill all kinds of insects, including those that had for centuries threatened the health of humans. One of its first major successes was in Naples in 1944, when that newly recaptured city was in the grip of an outbreak of typhus. The allied forces drafted in supplies of DDT to kill the lice that spread the disease.

DDT had first been made in 1874, by a chemistry student Othmer Zeidler, but its remarkable insecticidal activity went unnoticed. This was discovered in 1939 at the Geigy company in Switzerland, when Paul Herman Müller was searching for new insecticides. He realised that DDT offered benefits over the insecticides then in use, which were often based on lead and arsenic. They were known to be health hazards, but tests with DDT showed that it was not toxic to mammals. Müller received a Nobel Prize for his work in 1948.

DDT was eventually to save millions of human lives. It was responsible for eradicating the malaria-carrying mosquitos from the USA. It even wiped them out on the island of

Sri Lanka, after spraying began in every home there in 1948, when there were 2.5 million cases of the disease annually. By 1962 there were only 31 reported cases. But while the scourge of this ancient disease had apparently been lifted, concerns were being voiced over the build-up of DDT in the food chain. People were beginning to realise that it was adversely affecting some rare species of wildlife, such as the golden eagle. Most worrying of all, some species of insects were becoming resistant to it. Spraying in Sri Lanka was stopped, the mosquito returned, and soon the Sri Lankan doctors were again dealing with over two million cases of malaria a year.

Millions of tons of DDT were sprayed on crops each year, and it got into food as a contaminant. It began to accumulate in humans, and by the time DDT was phased out in the early 1970s, the average person had about 7 p.p.m. in their fatty tissues. Human metabolism deals with DDT by removing one of its chlorine atoms, and the metabolite thus formed is DDE, dichlorodiphenylethylene. This process is slow, and DDT has a half life in the body of 16 weeks. However, such levels were never dangerous to human health, and the WHO guidelines for a safe intake is 225 mg per year—about ten times the amount that consumers were exposed to when DDT use was at a maximum in the late 1960s.

DDT and PCBs are regarded by some agencies as potential carcinogens, a point made in a report from the US National Cancer Institute in 1993:

> Organochlorines such as DDT ... and PCBs ... which have been used extensively as insecticides and as fluid insulators of electrical components, respectively, are known to be persistent environmental contaminants and animal carcinogens. These agents have been found in human tissue due to their inefficient metabolism and their solubility in lipids .... Their association with human cancer occurrence, however, has been explored only marginally, with most studies having 20 or fewer cases.

One attempt to investigate the cancer-causing properties of organochlorines was a double-blind study designed to determine whether PCBs and/or DDE are associated with breast cancer in women. Blood samples of 14 290 participants, who enrolled between 1985 and 1991 in the New York University Women's Health Study, were analysed for PCBs and DDE using the technique known as gas chromatography. Women who were diagnosed with breast cancer had higher levels of DDE and PCBs than women who did not have the disease, but the differences were statistically significant only for DDE. Taking into account such factors as family history of breast cancer, lifetime lactation, and age at first full-term pregnancy, the analysis showed a fourfold increase in relative risk of breast cancer for those having most DDE in their serum. For PCBs, the relative risk was much less, and considering these same women also had DDE in their blood, it was concluded that for the women in this study, breast cancer could be associated with DDE in serum, but not with PCBs.

So organochlorine compounds have had a chequered history: while synthetic varieties have proved extremely useful, and natural ones are impossible to avoid, their impact on our health remains only poorly understood. While most people now accept that DDT, for example, is a threat to wildlife, there is little compelling evidence that it causes human cancer, as was once claimed. Elizabeth Whelan, president of the American Council on Science and Health, debates the pros and cons of DDT in her book *Toxic Terror*, and goes as far as to question the wisdom of banning this cheap and effective insecticide. Only time will tell if organochlorine chemicals pose a long-term threat. Meanwhile every effort is being made to find safer substitutes, to reduce the use of existing ones, and to dispose of them safely.

Information from many different sources indicates that the environment is becoming more polluted, and we know from past experience that these pollutants will end up in our food and drink. The effects of the non-nutrients mentioned in this chapter are being carefully monitored, and most of them offer no short-term danger. What they are doing in the long term is another matter. The unchecked manufacture of dangerous chemicals and the dumping of hazardous waste are now strictly controlled in the Western World, but in other countries priorities are very different, as people struggle to industrialise. We must be on guard to ensure that the increasing amount of food exported from these regions is not contaminated with their industrial wastes.

CHAPTER 10
Food for a healthy lifestyle

In this book we have tried to separate the facts from the myths that surround the food we eat. By now you will know how to avoid dangerous excesses of certain non-nutrients and how to keep clear of some of them altogether. You may also be reassured by the knowledge that, although there are risks in our food, they are not as alarming as some would have you believe.

To end this book it seems only right to offer some positive advice about diet. In this chapter we concentrate on what we feel are the most important aspects of healthy eating. A general guide to nutrition is to be found in Appendix 1.

If you are overweight, then the first piece of advice is that you should lose your excess body fat so that your weight falls in the range best suited to your height. The guideline that is most useful for determining whether you are overweight is the Body Mass Index (BMI), which is easily calculated: take your weight in kilograms and divide it by the square of your height in metres. You should get a value between 20 and 25: below 20 and you should put on weight; over 25 and you should lose it.

The average person weighing 70 kg and of height 1.7 metres has a BMI of 70 divided by 2.89 (i.e. 1.7×1.7), which comes to 24.2 and means they are OK. If you prefer to work in pounds and inches then divide your weight in pounds by the square of your height in inches, and multiply the result by 700. For example, if you are five feet six inches tall (66 inches) and weigh 150 pounds, then your BMI is 150 divided by 66×66, which comes to 0.0344, and this multiplied by 700 gives you a healthy BMI of 24. If you are this same height and you weigh 180 pounds, then your BMI is an unhealthy 29.

The next piece of advice that is given to those whose weight is about right, who don't smoke, and who take regular exercise, is to eat five portions of fruit or vegetables every day. This commonly offered advice is rarely explained, and here we offer some sound reasons for trying to stick to such a regime. Fruit and vegetables provide lots of useful carbohydrate, fibre, and vitamins; they can also provide protein and minerals as well.

And while none of the nutrients in food is specifically destined for the heart muscle, there are components that can ensure that this vital organ is not put at risk through dietary neglect. These components are also to be found in fresh fruit and vegetables.

The homocysteine saga: folate, B_6, and B_{12}

An important risk factor for disease of the circulatory system is raised levels in the blood of a body chemical called homocysteine, which is the breakdown product of the amino acid methionine. The body disposes of homocysteine as quickly as possible because it attacks the lining of the blood vessels. Yet a large number of people have elevated blood levels of homocysteine, because they have a deficiency of one or more of the vitamins that are co-factors for the enzymes that remove the unwanted homocysteine. These vitamins are folate, vitamin B_6, and vitamin B_{12}. Unfortunately in many people the gene that codes for the enzyme methylenetetrahydrofolate reductase, which recycles homocysteine back into methionine, produces a version that is less efficient at its job, and so more homocysteine stays for longer in their blood. Other people who have a rare genetic disorder called homocystinuria have so much homocysteine in their body that some is even excreted in their urine. All of these people are at increased risk of peripheral vascular, cardiovascular, and cerebrovascular diseases, which they experience as pain in the legs when walking, heart attacks, and strokes.

Homocystinuria sufferers develop cardiovascular diseases early in life, and as long ago as 1969 Kilmer McCully suggested that the raised levels of homocysteine in their blood were responsible. We now know that this is so: recently researchers at St Bartholomew's and the Royal London School of Medicine and Dentistry confirmed the link between homocysteine and ischemic heart disease, and recommended an increased consumption of folate to lower this risk. Similar research at university hospitals in Sri Lanka and Norway came to the same conclusion.

Animal studies have shown that homocysteine is a potent inducer of atherosclerosis, causing visible vascular damage within a week of continuous administration. Numerous studies have documented the association between occlusive vascular disease (narrowing of the arteries of the heart) and elevated blood levels of homocysteine. It has been estimated that the risk of this disease happening prematurely is about 30 times as great for people with higher levels of homocysteine, compared to individuals whose levels of this chemical are normal and low.

It is also known that people with the highest levels of homocysteine in their blood plasma (the top 5%) are more than three times as likely to suffer a heart attack than those with normal levels. This increased risk is in addition to the many other risk factors predisposing an individual to coronary heart disease, such as old age, diabetes, high blood pressure, being overweight, smoking, and high cholesterol levels.

Recently J. Selbub and colleagues, at the Human Nutrition Research Center on Aging, at Tufts University in Boston, USA, studied levels of plasma homocysteine and the vitamins involved in homocysteine metabolism in 1160 elderly people (67–96 years old) who had taken part in the earlier Framingham Heart Study. The Tufts researchers found that plasma homocysteine concentrations were adversely affected by lack of folate and vitamins B_6 and B_{12}. In other words, homocysteine levels went up when the intake of these vitamins was low, and this inverse relationship was linked to blood levels of folate, B_6, and B_{12}, and with the dietary intakes of folate and B_6. According to Selhub, prevention of this kind of vitamin deficiency in old age could lower the risk of vascular disease, which is the most common cause of death in the elderly. He suggested that folate, vitamin B_{12}, and vitamin B_6 were a necessary part of the diet in people over the age of 65 years. His report was published in the *Journal of the American Medical Association* in 1993, and it shows that, even including subjects who supplemented their diet with vitamins, only about 80% of those studied were consuming the current dietary reference value (DRV) of folate, which is 200 micrograms (µg) per day.

Folate (folic acid) (DRV 200 µg)

Folate is essential for the formation of red blood cells, and for growth and cell division. It prevents tissue dysplasia—a condition in which cells reproduce abnormally, and which is often a forerunner of cancer. There is also evidence that folate helps prevent coronary artery disease.

Folate is absorbed from the gastrointestinal tract and stored in the liver. Excess folate has no toxic effects, but deficiency causes anaemia, a sore, red, smooth tongue, disturbance of the intestinal tract, and poor growth in children. Folate deficiency is one of the most common vitamin deficiencies, and is likely to be a problem with the elderly and in pregnant women.

Since folate has a key role in the division of cells and growth, it is particularly important to ensure a regular supply during pregnancy and infancy. In pregnancy folate is also thought to protect the fetus against neural tubular defect, a defect when the two sides of the body fuse *in utero* and fail to do so completely, leading to conditions such as spina bifida, and women who are contemplating pregnancy are advised to take a supplement of 400 µg a day before they conceive, and to continue this up until the twelfth week of their pregnancy.

According to an article by William Willey and Meir Stampfer in the *Journal of the American Medical Association* (1993), the DRV for folate was until recently around 400 µg

Table 10.1 Folate in foods (DRV 200 µg).

Food (portion size)	Folate (µg)
Brewer's yeast (10 g)	400
Liver, lambs (100 g)	240
Spinach (100 g)	196
Potatoes (150 g)	145
Brussels sprouts (100 g)	110
Asparagus (100 g)	98
Broccoli (100 g)	65
Cauliflower (100 g)	50

per day, should probably be restored to that level from its current recommended level of 200 µg. Folate is cheap, readily available, and without any toxic side effects, so Willey and Stampfer's advice can easily be followed (see Table 10.1).

In a study of more than 5000 Canadians, blood folate levels were measured as part of a national nutrition survey conducted between 1970 and 1972. The people were then contacted 15 years later to see who had developed heart disease. The principal finding was that people with the lowest folate levels are at a 70% higher risk of dying from a heart attack compared to people with high folate levels.

Despite the benefits of folate, there is evidence that many people have very little of it in their diet. This vitamin is commonly found in a wide range of foods, but it is susceptible to both storage and cooking, which can lead to quite considerable depletion. Vegetables stored at room temperature slowly lose folate, but those stored in a refrigerator will show virtually no losses after two weeks. Further losses occur if the vegetables are exposed to light, so the best advice is to store them in the fridge, or at least in a dark pantry.

Vitamin B_6 (chemical name: pyridoxine) (DRV 1.4 mg men, 1.2 mg women

Vitamin B_6 plays an important role in the metabolism of fats, carbohydrates, and proteins. Toxicity is rare, but deficiency causes oily scaly skin, sore red tongue, loss of weight, irritability, and muscular weakness. In infants a lack of vitamin B_6 manifests itself in the form of diarrhoea, anaemia, and seizures. Vitamin B_6 is stored in quite high quantities in the liver, but it is important to maintain these levels so a daily intake is required. Table 10.2 lists the common foods that contain a lot of this vitamin.

The DRV for B_6 may be too low for certain individuals, such as pregnant and nursing mothers, women taking contraceptive pills, people on high protein diets, and the elderly. Half the people in the Selbub study (mentioned above, p. 137) showed B_6 dietary intakes below the DRV; and a large proportion of elderly people do not consume adequate B_6 as judged by the DRV standards, or by the impact that these vitamins should be having on the body's homocysteine.

Table 10.2 Vitamin B_6 in foods (DRV 1.4 mg men, 1.2 mg women).

Food (portion size)	Vitamin B_6 (mg)
Muesli (1 bowl, 95 g)	1.5
Bran flakes (1 bowl, 45 g)	0.8
Sunflower seeds (50 g)	0.6
Potatoes (150 g)	0.5
Avocado pear (half)	0.4
White fish (100 g)	0.3
Tuna, canned (100 g)	0.3
Banana (medium)	0.3
Peanuts (100 g)	0.3

The mysterious disappearance of vitamin B$_6$

Early in December 1952, the US Food and Drug Administration (FDA) received a letter from an Arkansas resident, a trained nurse, whose three-month-old infant was suffering from convulsive seizures. She gave a complete and informative case history of her child, who had been fed from birth on SMA liquid, a well-known brand of formula feed. The doctor who attended her baby suspected the condition was associated with the formula feed, and he changed the baby's diet to evaporated milk. The child recovered completely.

Through January and February of 1953, the FDA came across many more cases of what was now being called 'SMA convulsions'. These distressing attacks could last as long as five minutes, and the affected infants also displayed hyper-irritability, sensitivity to noise, diarrhoea, and vomiting. Doctors had prescribed various medications for the afflicted infants but the only thing which worked was a change of diet.

What puzzled the investigators was that only babies raised on SMA liquid were affected; no baby raised on powdered SMA suffered from convulsions. Yet both products were made from exactly the same ingredients. The FDA investigators were at a loss to understand what was going on, and in March 1953, they passed their files to the Division of Nutrition for study, asking if they could find an explanation. This was soon forthcoming.

The answer lay in research that had already been undertaken in the division's own laboratories. The babies' irritability and convulsive seizures resembled the symptoms shown by rats born to mothers on a vitamin B$_6$ deficient diet. When the young rats were given B$_6$ supplements they recovered, just as did the babies whose diet was changed. For some reason SMA liquid was deficient in vitamin B$_6$—but why?

The answer lay in the sterilisation process used to manufacture SMA liquid. At the raised temperatures that were used, the vitamin B$_6$ reacted chemically with amino acids and sugars in the milk to form compounds which a baby's metabolism could not use.

The manufacturing process, designed to ensure that SMA liquid would not be contaminated with disease organisms, had inadvertently converted the essential vitamin B$_6$ to a worthless non-nutrient.

The manufacturer of SMA liquid then started to add vitamin B$_6$ to their product, and within a few months there were no further cases of 'SMA convulsions'.

In the story in the box the devastating effects on this vitamin when milk is processed are illustrated in baby feed, but other processes lead to its loss as well. More than 75% may be removed during the milling of wheat for white flour, and currently there are no enrichment programmes in place to replace it. Freezing meat and poultry does not reduce their vitamin content, but it does with vegetables, and so does canning. However, subsequent storage does not seem to lead to any further losses. Cooking affects fruits, vegetables, and meat, with losses of B$_6$ as high as 50%.

Table 10.2 shows that there are plenty of cheap sources of vitamin B_6, such as bran flakes, potatoes, and tuna.

Excess vitamin B_6 Many people give themselves large daily doses of vitamin B_6 for a variety of reasons—but how much should be taken? In 1998 a UK Government committee called the Committee on Toxicity (COT) of Chemicals in Food, Consumer Products and the Environment reported on this, saying that people were overdosing on B_6, and recommended that over-the-counter sales of B_6 should provide for a daily dose of 10 mg per day. This was far lower that the dose that many people were already taking to relieve the symptoms of premenstrual tension, carpal tunnel syndrome (a wrist condition caused by repetitive strain injury), and morning sickness.

According to the consumer organisation, Consumers for Health Choice, around 3 million people in the UK were already taking 200 mg per day of B_6. However, another Government committee, the Agriculture Select Committee, criticised the COT recommendations and proposed that the limit should be set at 100 mg per day, in line with a report from the US National Academy of Sciences, which said that there was little evidence that even double this daily dose had a harmful effect.

However, excessive intake of vitamin B_6 has been known to cause sensory neuropathy, and this has been observed in women who were taking megadoses of as much as 2 g a day, which is more than 1600 times the DRV. The nerve damage this caused was totally cured when they stopped taking these excessive doses.

Vitamin B_{12} (chemical names: cobalamin or cyanocobalamin) (DRV 1.5 µg)

Vitamin B_{12} is important for the formation of red blood cells, the maintenance of nerve tissue, and the metabolism of carbohydrates, fats, and proteins to extract their energy. It is also needed to control pernicious anaemia.

Vitamin B_{12} is stored in the liver, which can hold up to five years' supply; however, regular intake is necessary to maintain this store. Vegan vegetarians have diets that are deficient in vitamin B_{12}, but this is not likely to be the case with diets that include meat and dairy produce.

No toxic effects are recorded from an excess of the vitamin. Symptoms of deficiency are a sore tongue, weakness, loss of weight, mental and nervous abnormalities, and back pain.

It has been said that anything that walks, swims, or flies contains vitamin B_{12}, whereas nothing that grows out of the ground needs this vitamin. Table 10.3 bears this out (see p. 142). Vitamin B_{12} is destroyed by light, and therefore shelf-lives of foods rich in it should be short if the maximum value is to be obtained. All forms of storage affect the vitamin a little, but the presence of vitamin C protects it. Unfortunately canning, and dehydrating remove this protection by destroying most of the vitamin C. Cooking will deplete vitamin B_{12} in all foods by about 40%. Pasteurization will only deplete milk by 10%, but evaporation of milk will destroy the B_{12} almost completely. Nevertheless, there are some easily obtained foods that contain more than enough to provide a week's supply of this vitamin, such as canned sardines.

Table 10.3 Vitamin B_{12} in foods (DRV 1.5 µg).

Food (portion size)	Vitamin B_{12} (µg)
Clams (100 g)	98.2
Liver, beef (100 g)	80.1
Pilchards (100 g)	12.0
Sardines (70 g)	10.0
Tuna (100 g)	4.2
Roast meat (100 g)	1.9
Eggs (2)	1.5
White fish (100 g)	1.0–3.0

'Take 5'

Pregnant women, and those who are planning to become pregnant, must ensure that their intake of folate is adequately maintained. A daily dose of 400 µg is recommended, because folate reduces the risk of neural tube defects in the fetus by about 70%. Other people, of both sexes and all ages, are not under the same imperative, and many of us are likely to be deficient in folate—but there is a simple way to remedy this. The long-forgotten advice of early nutritionists, to eat lots of fruit and vegetables every day, was sound advice indeed, and we would do well to heed it again. Five servings of fruits or vegetables per day should provide enough folate to prevent high levels of homocysteine, and there are indications that such a regime will also help prevent colon polyps, colon cancer, and cervical cancer.

Table 10.4 What constitutes a 'portion' of fruit or vegetable.

Apple, pear, banana, orange	1 whole fruit
Pineapple, melon	1 large slice
Plums, kiwi fruit, satsumas	2 whole fruits
Grapes, cherries, strawberries, raspberries	1 cupful
Canned fruits, fruit salad	3 tablespoonsful
Stewed fruit, prunes	3 tablespoonsful
Dried fruits (currants, raisins, figs, dates, etc.)	1 tablespoonful
Fruit juice	1 glass (150 ml)
All vegetables* (raw, cooked, frozen, canned)	2 tablespoonsful
Salad	1 dessert bowlful
Tomatoes	1 large, 2 medium, 4 small

*Except potatoes—see the text.

What exactly constitutes a 'portion' of fruit or of a vegetable? Table 10.4 gives some general guidance. Note that the table does not include potatoes, because these are regarded as primarily a source of starchy carbohydrate, so a portion of French fries or chips ought always to be accompanied by some other vegetable. Also note that the table does not include fruits high in oils such as olives and avocados, which are also excluded from the 'take 5' advice.

People who eat five servings of fruit or vegetables per day would not benefit from supplements, but as many fail to meet this intake, then vitamin supplementation to the DRV level of 200 µg is likely to be beneficial for the vast majority, and in particular for elderly people and women of childbearing age.

Fortunately, the simple rule of eating five pieces of fruit or portions of vegetables every day is easily obeyed, and all we may need to do is finish each meal with a piece of fruit to achieve the magic number.

Because so many Americans do not get enough folate in their diet, there is now a movement in the USA to fortify some common foods with it. In 1993 the US government legislated to fortify grain products with folate, and today it is available in foods such as bread, pasta, and cereal. According to researchers at the University of Washington, fortification offers the greatest potential for reducing coronary heart disease. Work done at Oregon's Regional Primate Research Center, at Beaverton, USA, and published in *The New England Journal of Medicine* in 1998, showed that breakfast cereals could reduce homocysteine levels by up to 14% provided they were fortified with folic acid. However, other researchers pointed out in an article in the *Journal of the American Medical Association* that fortification is expected to increase the intake of folic acid by only 100 µg per day, which would still leave about three quarters of the population with less than the 400 µg that these researchers think is necessary for maximum health benefit.

Even with raw foodstuffs, however, there may be less of these nutrients than we would like, because changes in agricultural production, transport, and storage may lead to some being lost. Further depletion may occur in food processing, from milling to canning, and finally the way we store and cook our food at home may make things worse. The major nutrients—carbohydrates, fats, and protein—are not generally reduced in all this, although their relative proportions can be altered in processed foods. It is the minor nutrients, and especially the micronutrients, that may be badly affected. Of these, selenium plays an important role in the health of our hearts.

Selenium (DRV 75 µg men, 60 µg women)

Selenium is a rare non-metallic element that is essential to the body in trace amounts. Unfortunately, due to modern farming methods, there is often insufficient selenium in the food chain, and on some selenium-deficient soils this element is now being added to fertilisers. Losses tend to occur in processing, such as in the milling of grain into flour, but cooking does not appear to cause serious depletion. The selenium that is present in the diet, in foods such as nuts, fish, and mushrooms (see Table 10.5), is easily absorbed from the intestine. Other factors in the diet will interfere with the absorption of selenium: high levels of fat and protein can reduce uptake.

Selenium, is given much more prominence today than in the past. Indeed, until the 1980s this little-known element was not thought to be a necessary part of human metabolism. Since then things have changed, and selenium is important enough to merit special mention when advice about improving one's diet is given.

Selenium may be a rare trace element, but it is essential to humans. It was proved to be a vital micronutrient in 1973, when it was discovered in the enzyme glutathione peroxidase

Table 10.5 Selenium in foods (DRV 75 µg men, 60 µg women).

Food (portion size)	Selenium (µg)
Brazil nuts (10 kernels)	200
Cashews (100 g)	67
White fish (150 g)	30–50
Wholemeal bread (2 slices)	30
Liver (100 g)	22
Pork (100 g)	15
Mushrooms (70 g)	8.5

which is responsible for reducing the dangerous hydroperoxides that form in cells, and can cause damage if not removed. In 1991 Dietrich Behne, in Berlin, found selenium in a second enzyme, deiodinase, which is involved in hormone production in the thyroid gland.

We need selenium only in microgram (µg) quantities, which is why it is classed as a micronutrient, but even so every cell of our body contains over a million selenium atoms. How much selenium the body needs, how much it takes in each day, and how much is excreted can vary within quite wide margins. It may be that a daily dose of 10 µg is enough, provided we get it every day; however, on some days we can lose more selenium than this.

Most selenium in the body is locked up in the bones rather than in soft tissue, but it does tend to accumulate in the hair, kidneys, and testicles. The average adult contains about 15 000 µg (15 mg, or a two thousandth part of an ounce). Yet to take this amount in as a single dose would be dangerous, and if we were to take in 50 mg at one go we could put our life at risk. However, amounts of selenium of this size are not associated with dietary intake, only with accidental poisoning or industrial exposure. Excess selenium can be removed from the body in the urine and faeces and also through the lungs and sweat glands as vile smelling volatile selenium compounds. The characteristic symptoms of selenium poisoning are easily recognised as terrible body odour and bad breath. To avoid poisoning, the recommended maximum daily intake of selenium is 0.45 mg (450 µg). For good health, the DRV is 60 µg for an adult woman and 75 µg for an adult man.

If the amount of selenium in our body is too low then we are at risk from a range of conditions such as anaemia, high blood pressure, infertility, cancer, arthritis, premature ageing, muscular dystrophy, and multiple sclerosis. There is no scientific proof that selenium will prevent these conditions, but there is some epidemiological evidence that it can protect us against them. It can certainly protect us against toxic metals such as mercury, cadmium, arsenic, and lead. This may explain why tuna fish, which accumulate small amounts of mercury from the marine environment, are not affected by it: they accumulate selenium as well.

Those most at risk of selenium deficiency are pregnant and breast-feeding women, and children, but they would have to eat a very strange diet if they were to avoid selenium altogether. Plants produced in certain parts of the world are almost completely devoid of selenium because the soil they are grown in has very little of it, and this may adversely affect livestock as well as people. The converse is also true: some areas are rich in selenium and plants absorb so much that they become poisonous to the animals that eat them.

Consequently it is rather difficult to make recommendations for selenium levels in animal feeds, and researchers in the USA have shown that a supplement of just 0.1 p.p.m. to an animal's diet can lead to a 70% increase in the selenium content of beef liver.

In people, daily intake can be as low as 6 µg and as high as 200 µg, depending on their diet. The average western diet will provide about 60 µg per day, which is more than enough to prevent the symptoms of selenium deficiency in a woman but slightly less than required by a man. Most of us get our daily dose of selenium from breakfast cereals and bread, but there are much richer sources of this element, and the following have levels in excess of 30 µg per 100 g: seafoods, such as tuna, cod, and salmon; offal, such as liver and kidney; nuts, such as Brazil nuts, cashew nuts, and peanuts; and wheat germ, bran, and brewer's yeast. Selenium supplements come in the form of sodium selenite, which is a white crystalline material that is soluble in water, and the suggested daily dose taken this way is 50 µg.

Selenium was first popularised by Alan Lewis in his book *Selenium: the Essential Trace Element You Might Not be Getting Enough of*, which was published in 1982. He argued that selenium could ward off arthritis, heart disease, cancer and other symptoms of old age, but it is unlikely that selenium can offer all of these benefits. However, research in China did reveal that a lack of selenium was the cause of a rare heart disease. It had long been known that children in the Keshan region of China were liable to suffer a heart condition known as Keshan disease, which causes an abnormal swelling of the heart and kills half of those afflicted. In 1974 a large-scale trial in southern China involved 20 000 children, half of whom were given tablets containing selenium and half were given a placebo. Of those on the placebo, 106 developed Keshan disease and 53 died, while of those taking the selenium supplement only 17 got Keshan and one died.

Also in China, other large-scale experiments in the 1980s found selenium was beneficial in reducing the incidence of various types of cancer. People living in the north central province of Linxian suffered a high incidence of stomach cancer. They agreed to take part in a five-year project and 30 000 middle-aged people were given different combinations of vitamins A, B_2, C, E, zinc, and selenium. The study showed a remarkably reduced incidence of cancer in the group taking vitamin E plus selenium.

In another study to see whether selenium could slow the development of skin cancer, 500 people with this condition were given a daily dose of 200 µg of selenium, while a control group received no extra selenium. Taking the selenium supplements for 5–6 years did not affect the rate of recurrence of skin cancer, but it did reduce the incidence of lung, colorectal, and prostate cancers. If this study can be confirmed in a larger group of people, it is likely that selenium will one day be added to flour used to make cereals and breads. But consuming sufficient fruit and vegetables (good sources of selenium and folic acid) instead of refined flour would be equally good, according to the *Journal of the American Medical Association* (1996).

Selenium has recently become accepted as having a key role in fertility. This was made clear in 1993, when the Scottish researcher Alan MacPherson reported on a double-blind, placebo-controlled trial using selenium supplementation. This research revealed that men whose sperm counts were low, and who were given selenium, showed an increase in sperm quality of 100%.

In 1997 Dr Margaret P. Ryman wrote an editorial in the *British Medical Journal* in which she said that the problems most associated with low selenium levels are infertility, cancer, and heart disease. She claimed that declining sperm quality and increased incidence of cancer could be explained by the fall in intake of selenium: in England, the average intake declined by half in the course of the last quarter of the twentieth century. The same was true in the Scandinavian countries and in the rest of Europe.

Clearly, selenium deserves more attention than it has received. In the UK, farmers have been giving their animals selenium supplements for years to keep them healthy, and Ryman noted the irony that nobody has suggested a similar policy for humans. She even suggested that governments should adopt measures like those adopted in Finland in 1984, when a programme for selenium enrichment of the soil through selenium-enhanced fertilisers was put into operation. While this would provide a long-term solution to the problem of selenium-deficient foods from selenium-deficient soils, a more immediate solution would be to fortify various foodstuffs with this micronutrient. Meanwhile, we should encourage people to eat more Brazil nuts, which are the best food source of selenium, or to take a daily selenium supplement.

The ACE vitamins

One theory of ageing is that as we grow older we can no longer repair all the damage that free radicals cause within our bodies. Free radicals are molecules that have a rogue electron, and it is this which gives them the ability to attack anything they come across. Free radicals are implicated in all kinds of cell damage, including damage to the DNA. This can produce mutant DNA, which if it is not recognised could lead to cancer. Several other health problems have been blamed on free radicals: heart disease, nerve damage, immunity weakness, and arthritis, although *proving* that this is the cause is another matter.

The production of free radicals comes as a consequence of our body needing oxygen in large amounts, mainly so that it can react with molecules such as glucose, to provide warmth, motion, and the energy to fuel the hundreds of chemical reactions that we need to keep our body working. Oxygen gas is itself a free radical, with *two* rogue electrons, which suggests it would be doubly dangerous, but it is a curious property of this element that it is much more stable than most other free radicals, and stable enough to have built up in the atmosphere over hundreds of millions of years until it accounts for around 20% of the air that we breath.

Oxygen is taken in to our lungs and there passes to the haemoglobin of our blood, which can transport it to wherever it is needed in the body. As it reacts with other components it forms other free radicals, and these are the dangerous ones. Fortunately our body has its defenders ready, and these are anti-oxidant molecules, metals, and enzymes such as super-oxide dismutase, that will 'quench' the fire of the free radicals. Components in food are capable of acting as anti-oxidants, such as the polyphenols of tea and red wine, which were mentioned on pages 21 and 76, and even some food additives may help in this respect. The sulfur molecules that give garlic its distinctive odour are also thought to have excellent anti-oxidant properties. Butyl hydroxytoluene (BTH), which is added to oils, and foods based on such oils, to prevent them going rancid, may even protect us against free radicals, for the same reason that it protects the oils: it guards against attack by oxygen.

The most efficient antioxidants are the vitamins A, C, and E. While these vitamins have several roles to play in keeping us healthy, their anti-oxidant activity means that we should try and maintain a regular supply of them in our diet.

Vitamin A (chemical names: retinol, carotene) (DRV 700 μg men, 600 μg women)

Vitamin A is required to maintain normal vision at night, and it is essential for successful calcium absorption for healthy body, tooth, and bone growth. It also maintains the linings of the nose, the throat, the respiratory and digestive systems, and the genito-urinary tract. Deficiency of vitamin A causes night blindness, stunted growth, and abnormal teeth in children, rough scaly skin, sore throats, increased susceptibility to sinus infections, abscesses of the mouth and ears, diarrhoea, and kidney and bladder disorders.

Vitamin A is provided by foods such as dairy products, eggs, and liver, which contain the chemical beta-carotene. This beta-carotene is absorbed not in the stomach, but in the small intestine, where it is mixed with fats and bile salts and converted into vitamin A. Excess of vitamin A can be stored in the liver, and released into the blood as required. Healthy adults with a good intake of beta-carotene can store enough vitamin A to meet the body's requirement for up to a year. Excessive intake of beta-carotene in the diet can not cause poisoning, but it may cause a yellow discoloration of the skin which disappears when the excess is reduced.

Vitamin A and beta-carotene are insoluble in water and are not affected by boiling, so normal cooking does not leach them out of food, nor destroy them. Canning reduces beta-carotene, and therefore canned vegetables do not provide us with as much vitamin A as fresh vegetables. Exposure to ultraviolet light destroys vitamin A, so foods that are rich in it should be stored in the dark, and consumed as soon as possible after harvest or slaughter. Because of its intense heat, barbecuing will destroy a lot of the vitamin A in food. Table 10.6 lists common foods that have the highest levels of this vitamin.

Table 10.6 Vitamin A in foods (DRV 700 μg men, 600 μg women).

Food (portion size)	Vitamin A (μg)
Liver, calf, cooked (100 g)	40 000
Liver sausage (100 g)	2 500
Butter (100 g)	830
Double cream (50 g)	570
Cheddar cheese (100 g)	320
Whole milk (half pint)	150
Egg, medium (60 g)	110

Vitamin C (chemical name: ascorbic acid) (DRV 60 mg)

Vitamin C keeps gums healthy, strengthens capillary walls of blood vessels, helps wounds and burns to heal, and aids the absorption of vitamin A, iron, and folic acid. Excess vitamin C is excreted in the urine, producing an acidified urine, and this is likely to happen to those who regularly prescribe themselves megadoses of this vitamin, sometimes as much as 10 g a day. Too little vitamin C will cause loss of weight, listlessness, fatigue, joint and muscle pains, and sore and bleeding gums. Severe deficiency eventually leads to scurvy—a potentially fatal disease of internal bleeding that has caused untold misery down the centuries.

The first reports of scurvy came from Vasco da Gama during his voyage round the Cape of Good Hope in 1497: he lost 100 of his 160-strong crew to the disease. For the next 300 years scurvy was part of life on the high seas, and despite early recognition that citrus fruits could prevent it, there was no agreement as to its cause or treatment. Blame for the disease fell on foggy weather, salted food, rancid butter, copper pans, sugar, tobacco, laziness, and the time of year. Some of these were near the mark: copper pans destroy vitamin C by reacting with it chemically; and the disease was likely to appear in winter and early spring because stored foodstuffs slowly lose their vitamin C content. But even when the Royal Navy surgeon James Lind showed in 1747 what lemon juice could do in curing advanced cases of scurvy, his advice was not acted upon; and during the Seven Years War (1756–63), 130 000 British sailors died of the disease. One problem was that lemons were thought to work because of their acidity, so ships carried vinegar or even dilute sulfuric acid to treat the disease. When lemon juice itself was accepted as beneficial, it was often boiled and bottled to store it—processes that robbed it of most of its vitamin C.

It was only in the twentieth century that vitamin C was identified, and its effects on animals and humans noted. Guinea pigs, like humans, cannot make vitamin C, and have to take it in with their food. In 1907 Norwegian researchers Axel Holst and Theodor Frölich put guinea pigs on restricted diets, and noted that some of them went down with scurvy. In 1918 Harriette Chick at the Lister Institute, London, was able to identify foods that would prevent the disease in guinea pigs, and in 1919 the unknown component was labelled vitamin C (vitamins A and B had already been identified).

In 1928 the Hungarian biochemist Albert Szent-Györgyi isolated the chemical, and in 1933 Walter Norman Haworth worked out its molecular structure. The following year, the Swiss chemist Tadeus Reichstein made vitamin C synthetically. Today it is manufactured from glucose using the process that Reichstein devised, and every year 50 000 tonnes are produced worldwide. As well as being sold in tablet form, and taken by millions of people, it is also widely used as a food additive (its code is E300 in the European system), particularly in fruit drinks and other foods where the naturally occurring vitamin C may be depleted during food processing.

Vitamin C is found mainly in foods of plant origin, especially citrus fruits and potatoes (see Table 10.7). The amount depends on how and where the plants have been grown, and how long the foods have been stored. Plants that have been exposed in the growing stage to more sunshine will have a higher vitamin C content, and, for example, potatoes lose 75% of their vitamin C when stored for a few months. Because of their acidity, however, citrus fruits

Table 10.7 Vitamin C in foods (DRV 60 mg).

Food (portion size)	Vitamin C (mg)
Peppers, red, raw (50 g)	140
Peppers green, raw (50 g)	120
Brussels sprouts, cooked (100 g)	115
Blackcurrants, stewed (100 g)	115
Kiwi fruit, raw (100 g)	98
Orange juice (1 large glass)	80
Potatoes* (150 g)	26
Tomatoes, fresh (100 g)	17

*Boiled, baked, roasted, or fried.

have a natural ability to preserve their vitamin C. Table 10.7 lists common foods that are good sources.

Vitamin C is chemically unstable, and can react with many other components in food as well as be destroyed by heat, oxygen, enzymes, alkalis and copper atoms. Washing, soaking, and cutting food will reduce the amount of vitamin C, whereas steaming can help preserve it by destroying the enzymes that attack it. Least vitamin C is lost when food is quick-frozen, and most is lost when food is air-dried in sunlight.

Food manufacturers are aware of the damage processing can do to vitamin C and they can take action to replace any that is lost. On the other hand, cooks, whether at home, or in cafés and canteens, are likely to reduce the level of vitamin C in the food they prepare. They are best advised to buy fruit and vegetables in small quantities, and to use them when they are fresh.

Vitamin C is water soluble, and therefore is lost in cooking: for example, Brussels sprouts when freshly picked contain 230 mg of vitamin C per 100 g, but after cooking this has fallen to around 115 mg. Even so, a portion of this vegetable eaten with your meal can provide your daily requirement. But most foods have less vitamin C than Brussels sprouts, and so it is worth preserving it by cooking in small quantities of water, or, better still, steaming or broiling, and serving and eating immediately. Wherever possible, cook vegetables with their skins on, rather than peeling, chopping, and soaking them first; and do not leave frozen vegetable to thaw before cooking.

Vitamin E (chemical name: a–tocopherol) (DRV 10 mg)

Vitamin E strengthens the walls of blood capillaries, and surveys suggest that it may protect against heart disease and cancer. Deficiency of vitamin E is rare, because it is found in many foods (see Table 10.8) and stored in many tissues of the body. However, it is easily destroyed when food is processed, so foods containing vitamin E are best eaten as fresh as possible—they should not be fried, frozen, or canned, and storage times should be kept to a minimum. Unprocessed flour is better than white processed flour, which retains only 20% of the original content of vitamin E. This vitamin is not soluble in water, so very little is lost in cooking.

Table 10.8 Vitamin E in foods (DRV 10 mg).

Food (portion size)	Vitamin E (mg)
Almonds, shelled (100 g)	24.5
Cashews, dry roasted (100 g)	11
Sunflower oil (1 tablespoon)	10
Sweet potatoes (150 g)	6.5
Flour, whole-wheat (100 g)	3.9
Avocado (half)	3.0
Rice, brown (100 g)	2.0

Summing up

There has long been a tendency to greet each new dietary discovery as the key to a healthier and longer life. As the importance of the various vitamins and minerals was realised, so there often appeared a popular book interpreting the discovery as a cure-all. Over the years there have been many such books, advocating diets rich in vitamin C, zinc, essential amino acids, fibre, magnesium, and unsaturated fats, or low in supposed dangers such as cholesterol. There are already books advocating selenium, and the temptation is to see this as yet another food fad that will come and go in the same way as all the others. Perhaps it will, but developments in food science are now much better grounded in nutrition, food chemistry, and medical research, and together these are achieving such successes that a healthy, but ageing, population is now seen as a 'problem' for the next century.

The advice given in this chapter is as well-founded, in scientific terms, as it is possible to be, and you would be well advised at least to try a diet that contains more fruit, vegetables, and selenium. Meanwhile, become alert to the hidden dangers in your diet, so you can decide if you experience food intolerances. If you do, you can adjust your eating habits accordingly, and enjoy your food into a rewarding old age.

Appendix 1:
A guide to nutrition

A great deal of research over the past century by food chemists, biochemists, and medical researchers has gone into determining what proportions and basic minimum intake of these different food components should be. For example, the UK's Committee on Medical Aspects of Food (COMA) advises that our daily intake of the major macronutrients should be roughly as follows: protein, 15%; carbohydrate, 55%; and fats, 30% (all by weight).

The primary reason why our body demands food several times a day is that we need energy. By oxidising our food, we generate warmth for our body and energy to do work. Fats, proteins, carbohydrates, and alcohol are all good sources of energy. Carbohydrates provide most of our daily needs; and though fats contain more energy, weight-for-weight, they take longer to digest and so release their energy over a longer period of time. The body can also break down protein and use that to generate energy, but this is generally done only when other sources of energy have been used up. If we have too many calories in our diet, combined with too little in the way of exercise, our body will store energy by making fat cells. In the long run this will cause obesity, with all its attendant problems: high blood pressure, heart disease, and sometimes diabetes.

Too few calories in our diet, and too much energy demanded of our bodies, will lead to loss of weight, as our body burns up its fatty tissues. When that reserve is used up, the body will convert muscle and other protein to energy. This will lead to tiredness and retarded growth and development, and it will make us more susceptible to illness. This is partly why diseases flourish at times of famine and food shortages, such as during natural disasters and wars. Nevertheless, an adult can recover from a period of enforced starvation and suffer little long-term damage; but for children starvation is soon fatal, and for teenagers it may do permanent damage.

Macronutrients
Protein

We need protein to make new body tissues. This process starts on the day we are conceived and goes on until the day we die. Even when we have stopped growing, we need to replace tissues as they become worn out. Blood cells, for example, last about 120 days, and the lining of the stomach and intestine needs replacing every 36 hours. Proteins are found throughout the body, and have many different functions. The cells of the body are surrounded by fluid containing proteins, and haemoglobin is a protein that picks up oxygen in the lungs and carries it round the body in the red blood cells. Other proteins are found in the plasma: they regulate the amount of water in the body, as well as acting as buffers to control the body's acid balance. Enzymes are proteins, and these are vital to carrying out numerous chemical reactions, including the joining together of amino acids to form other types of protein. Antibodies, which protect us against bacteria and viruses, are also proteins, and so are the agents responsible for the clotting mechanisms that stop bleeding.

Protein occurs naturally in all living things, and every different protein has a unique chemical structure and function determined by the DNA of the organism that produced it. Our proteins are made from amino acids according to the codes written into our genes, and because one amino acid or protein cannot be substituted for another in the body, we have to keep a good balance in our diet of all the amino acids that we need.

The proteins we take in as part of our food are digested by enzymes which first of all break them down into their constituent amino acids. These can then pass through the gut wall into the bloodstream, and be taken to where they are needed. We constantly lose the waste products from used protein in faeces, urine, perspiration, hair, and skin, and it needs to be replaced on a daily basis if we are to stay healthy. The recommended daily intake for a healthy person is at least 1 g per kilogram of body weight, and there is no difference between the needs of men and women. However, because men usually weigh more than women, their total intake has to be higher.

Not all dietary protein is of equal value, because some may be lacking in so-called *essential* amino acids that we need to make our own protein, and which we can only obtain from our diet. We can obtain the other amino acids from our food, but they can also be made in our bodies. The essential amino acids are isoleucine, leucine, lysine, methionine, phenylalanine, threonine, tryptophan, and valine. Gelatin is a protein but it would not sustain life if it was our only source of protein, because it is deficient in tryptophan which is essential for human tissue. In general, animal proteins are of more value as food than plant proteins, because they more closely reflect the spectrum of amino acids that we, as animals, need.

Foods high in protein are meats, fish, cheese, beans, eggs, nuts, and pulses. Table A1.1 lists the foods that supply most protein, together with their biological value. In the table 'high' means that the protein supplies all the amino acids the human body needs, 'medium' means that one of the essential amino acids is missing, and 'low' means that two or more are missing.

Carbohydrate (CHO)

Carbohydrates are organic compounds made up of carbon (C), hydrogen (H), and oxygen (O), and they are given the shorthand name CHO. Plants make carbohydrates from water and carbon dioxide, using the Sun's energy to convert these raw materials to CHO, and

Table A1.1 Foods with the highest protein content, and their biological value.

Food	Protein content (g/100 g)	Biological value	Missing amino acids
Soybean (dried)	36	high	none
Peanuts	26	low	lysine, methionine, threonine, tryptophan
Cheddar cheese	25	high	none
Lentils	24	medium	methionine
Kidney beans	22	medium	methionine
Cashew nuts	21	low	lysine, methionine
Almonds	21	low	lysine, methionine
Chicken	20	high	none
Fish	19	high	none
Beef	19	high	none

giving off oxygen gas. When we burn carbohydrates in a fire, e.g. as logs or leaves, we are simply reversing the process, reacting CHO with oxygen from the air, to form water and carbon dioxide. The same chemical reaction occurs in the cells of our body, but under more carefully controlled conditions. The end result is the same: warmth and energy to do work.

The carbohydrate in our food comes in many different forms such as sugar and starch. Our digestive enzymes break these larger molecules down into their constituent parts, which are mostly glucose molecules. The brain needs an endless supply of this particular carbohydrate. Glucose is easily absorbed into the body, where it can immediately be tapped for energy; or, if there is a surplus, it can be stored in the liver as glycogen. Glycogen is constantly being formed and changed back into glucose by the liver, so that the level of glucose in the blood remains between certain set limits. This ensures a more or less constant energy supply for our daily activity.

Not all carbohydrate is instantly digested. Some acts as fibre, and we will look at this beneficial non-nutrient later in this appendix.

There is no specific requirement for particular carbohydrates, and there is a wide variety that we can use. They are found in bread, potatoes, rice, pasta, fruits, vegetables, cereals, and milk. The world's major food crops—wheat, rice, potatoes, and maize—are all rich sources of carbohydrate.

Carbohydrates represent the most immditely available calories. Meeting the body's energy requirements takes precedence over anything else, and if the diet is lacking in carbohydrates, other sources of energy have to be found. This may mean breaking down body tissue to release amino acids for burning. At the other extreme, we may take in so much carbohydrate that the body continues to convert a lot of it to fat, even if we already have enough fat to sustain us through a period when food is in short supply.

The total CHO content of a particular food is the total of all the edible carbohydrates it contains, including starch and sugars such as sucrose (ordinary sugar), lactose (from milk), and fructose (which is common in many fruits). These sugars eaten in sensible quntities are useful nutrients. One sugar in particular is attractive to the human palate because of its sweetness, and that is sucrose. The current consumption of this as ordinary sugar accounts for as much as 10% of our daily calorie intake, because it is added to many processed foods including some that are not obviously sweet, such as savoury sauces.

Fat

Fat in the diet serves several important functions in the body. It provides linoleic acid, which is an essential fatty acid the body cannot manufacture for itself, but which is needed for building cells. Linoleic acid also contributes to a number of important chemical messengers such as the prostaglandins, which are involved in reproduction and the circulation. Fat is a source of energy, and it provides a convenient storage facility because it packs more energy into the same volume than any other chemical. It is responsible for body shape, particularly in women, and it acts as a layer of heat insulation beneath the skin. Fat in the diet may bring with it certain fat-soluble vitamins, such as vitamins A and D, and flavour molecules; and it also controls the rate at which food passes through the gut.

Fats and oils are the same kind of chemical, and are known technically as triglycerides. The difference between them is that fats are solid at room temperature, while oils are liquid. They are made from the same fatty acids, but in slightly different combinations. Some of these fatty acids are called 'saturated' and some 'unsaturated,' chemical terms that describe their molecular bonding—not how many calories they contain. Unsaturated fatty acids come in several types, which are described by terms such as 'monounsaturated,' 'polyunsaturated,' and 'trans fatty acids.'

Some dietary theories have been built around the benefits of avoiding saturated and trans-fatty acids, and concentrating on monounsaturated and polyunsaturated oils and fats. The foods highest in unsaturated fats are the vegetable oils, such as olive, sunflower, corn, rape-seed (canola), soya, and some nut oils (but not coconut oil which is the most saturated fat of all). The foods highest in saturated fats are dairy products and hard animal fats. To digest fat the body needs cholesterol, which is regarded by some as a hidden danger in our diet. In fact cholesterol is an essential body chemical, and it is found in all body tissues, the highest quantities being in the brain and spinal chord. It is a constituent of cell membranes, and particularly of the myelin sheath that protects nerves. It is a precursor of the bile acids that are needed to digest the food in our gut. And it is a precursor of steroid hormones, including the sex hormones and those that play a part in anti-stress mechanisms, water balance, and other metabolic processes. Most of our cholesterol is manufactured by the liver, but almost any tissue in the body is capable of making it. Our body can generate all the cholesterol it needs, but it can take in some from the food we eat. However, even if we eat foods rich in cholesterol, only a small fraction of it will get into our bloodstream.

Cholesterol is present in many foods, such as eggs, meat, poultry, dairy products, animal fats, oils, and fish. Food with very high levels are egg yolk, kidney, liver, butter, shrimps, fish roe, cream, hard cheeses, turkey, beef, and lamb. One of the highest levels is in the yolks of hens' eggs, which contain 1.2%. Plants have no need for cholesterol, so there are many foods that contain none at all. Indeed, vegan vegetarians, who live only on plant foods, take in no dietary cholesterol, and the 100 g of this chemical that is in their body tissue has all been made by their own metabolism.

High levels of cholesterol in the blood are considered to be unhealthy, and to increase the risk of coronary heart disease and strokes. If cholesterol levels are high, it may form fatty deposits on the walls of blood vessels, which, over a period of time, can become narrow, leading to heart disease and degeneration of the arteries. We can take some steps to control the amount of cholesterol in our body by reducing the amount of fat we eat, giving up smoking, maintaining the correct body weight, and taking regular exercise, although in some cases it is necessary to take medication as well.

Minerals

The minerals we need to take into our body in substantial amounts are calcium, magnesium, potassium, sodium, phosphate, and chloride. How much of these we need depends on our age and gender, but there are published guidelines to help us. For these six minerals the DRVs are: calcium 700 mg (for the average adult); magnesium 300 mg; potassium 3500 mg; sodium 1600 mg; phosphate 800 mg; and chloride 2500 mg. Chloride intake is closely linked to sodium intake, since the two come into the body together in the form of salt (sodium chloride). Few people suffer from deficiencies of these minerals; if anything, we tend to exceed these recommended amounts, often markedly so.

Calcium (DRV 700 mg) Calcium deficiency may be due to a low dietary intake, lack of vitamin D, lack of stomach acid, coeliac disease, or lactose intolerance. Those taking the contraceptive pill, corticosteroid drugs, or diuretic treatments may also have reduced calcium absorption. Pregnant and breast-feeding women may also lack calcium because of the requirements of the baby. Post menopausal women lose about 1% of bone density per year which is entirely due to a loss of calcium and which can be reversed by hormone replacement therapy.

Ideally the ratio of calcium to phosphate in the diet should be 1:1, and the amount of vitamin D should be adequate. Table A1.2 gives the calcium levels of foods particularly rich in this mineral.

Table A1.2 Calcium in foods (DRV 700 mg).

Food (portion size)	Calcium (mg)
Cheddar cheese, Edam cheese (50 g)	360
Sardines, canned (70 g)	350
Milk: whole, semi-skimmed, or skimmed (half pint)	350
Tofu (60 g)	300
Milk chocolate (100 g)	240

Magnesium (DRV 300 mg)
Magnesium is an important element in the body: it is necessary for the metabolism of calcium, phosphorus, sodium, potassium, and vitamin C. It is also essential for effective nerve and muscle functioning, and for converting glucose into energy.

Table A1.3 Magnesium in foods (DRV 300 mg).

Food (portion size)	Magnesium (mg)
Taco shells (100 g)	104
Muesli (1 bowl, 95 g)	90
Brazil nuts (10 kernels)	80
Baked beans (200 g)	60
Almonds (10 kernels)	50
Rice, brown (100 g)	35

The requirement for magnesium is easily met in a normal diet because many common foods provide it (see Table A1.3). Dairy products are particularly rich in magnesium. However, the refining and processing of grains and sugar reduces their magnesium content considerably, and cooking vegetables in large amounts of water leaches out their soluble magnesium. Also, alcohol and diuretics interfere with the body's ability to absorb and retain this mineral.

Potassium (DRV 3500 mg) Potassium, together with sodium, maintains the osmotic pressure that controls the passage of fluid into body cells, and it also ensures a proper acid–base balance of the blood and body tissues. It is essential in the functioning of muscle and nerves, and for the secretion of insulin by the pancreas. Potassium helps to transport oxygen to the brain, dispose of body wastes, and control blood pressure.

The most common foods with high levels of potassium are given in Table A1.4. Bananas, which are popularly thought of as rich in potassium, do have high levels: a large banana weighing 100 g (3½ ounces) would provide 350 mg. It is very difficult with a normal diet and healthy kidneys to overload the system with potassium—such overload is usually associated with severe illness. Nevertheless, potassium supplements should only be taken under the supervision of a physician.

Table A1.4 Potassium in foods (DRV 3500 mg).

Food (portion size)	Potassium (mg)
Vegetable curry (300 g)	1250
Potato crisps/Potato chips (100 g)	1190
Baked potato (150 g)	950
Cantaloupe melon (half)	750
Peanuts (100 g)	680
Tomato juice (large glass)	460
Milk chocolate (100 g)	420
Banana (100 g)	350

Sodium (DRV 1600 mg) Sodium plays the major part in maintaining the balance of water in our bodies. It is also a constituent of sweat, tears, and bile salts, and is needed to preserve muscle and nerve functions. Sodium is also involved in the absorption of carbohydrates in the diet. Most of our intake of sodium is in the form of added salt (sodium

Table A1.5 Sodium in foods (DRV 1600 mg).

Food (portion size)	Sodium (mg)
Crab, canned (100 g)	1000
Cheddar cheese (100 g)	700
Cornflakes (100 g)	660
Tomato puree (100 g)	590
Bread, white, 3 slices (100 g)	500

chloride), or as ingredients such as the sodium bicarbonate used in baking and sodium nitrate preservative in cooked meats: about a third of our intake comes from the sodium naturally present in our food. Sodium is readily absorbed in the gut, and it is then transported to the kidneys, where its level in the blood is adjusted before it is distributed around the body.

Bouts of severe vomiting, diarrhoea, profuse sweating can all cause depletion of sodium. But for most people, the problem is too much salt in their diet. Over a long period of time this can lead to high blood pressure, and swelling of the legs and face. So it is important to regulate the intake of dietary salt, which is easily done by not using too much while cooking, and not adding too much while eating. Many processed foods, such as bread, cornflakes, and savoury snacks, contain large quantities of salt, but since the salt is such an important component of their flavour it is unlikely it will ever be taken out. Salt suppresses bitterness in foods, which is why sprinkling it on grapefruit produces a much better flavour. Table A1.5 shows the sodium levels in various kinds of foods.

Phosphate (DRV 800mg) Phosphate plays a part in a variety of body structures and processes. Bone is primarily calcium phosphate, and there are many other phosphates, such as ATP (adenosine triphosphate) which is the energy molecule that drives many metabolic processes. DNA also contains phosphate.

Vegan vegetarians who take in no dairy foods are at risk, and there are certain diseases that interfere with phosphate metabolism. Prolonged intake of antacid medicines can also have an effect. However, all of these situations are rare, and most people absorb sufficient quantities of phosphate from their food.

Micronutrients

Micronutrients are the vitamins and minerals that we need only in milligram (mg) or microgram (µg) quantities. Table A1.6 gives the DRVs, or recommended daily allowances, of the micronutrients for the average person. This table is based on the *Dietary Reference Values for Food Energy and Nutrient for the United Kingdom*, and should only be used as a general guide: DRVs do not take into account people with special needs such as those suffering from an infection, those with inherited disorders of metabolism, and those with chronic diseases. These people's needs require professional assessment, and a variety of

Table A1.6 The DRVs for vitamins and minerals.

Micronutrient	Men	Women
Vitamins		
A	700 µg	600 µg
Thiamin (B₁)	1.0 mg	0.8 mg
Riboflavin (B₂)	1.3 mg	1.1 mg
Niacin	18 mg	13 mg
B₆ (pyridoxine)	1.4 mg	1.2 mg
B₁₂	1.5 µg	1.5 µg
Folate	200 µg	200 µg
Pantothenic acid*	3–7 mg	3–7 mg
Biotin* (see text)	10–200 µg	10–200 µg
C (see p. 148)	40 mg	40 mg
D* (see text)	10 µg	10 µg
E* (see p. 149)	10 mg	10 mg
K*	70 µg	70 µg
Minerals		
Iron	9 mg	15 mg
Copper	1.2 mg	1.2 mg
Zinc	10 mg	7 mg
Manganese*	above 1.4 mg	above 1.4 mg
Molybdenum*	50–400 µg	50–400 µg
Chromium*	above 25 µg	above 25 µg
Selenium	75 µg	60 µg
Iodine	140 µg	140 µg

*Suggested range, no DRV yet decided.

other factors, such as age, gender, height, weight, and physical activity have to be taken into consideration when micronutrient intake is being assessed.

Vitamins

Vitamin A See chapter 10, p. 147.

Thiamin (vitamin B₁) (DRV 1.0 mg men, 0.8 mg women) Thiamin (vitamin B₁) has many roles. It plays an important part in energy metabolism; it helps to keep the peripheral nerves healthy; it maintains a normal appetite; it aids degestion, especially of carbohydrates; it produces good muscle tone; and it engenders a healthy mental attitude to life.

Only small amounts of thiamin are stored in the body—about enough to meet the body's full needs for a week. It is important to keep up the supply because in times of illness great demands are made. Thiamin is found in a variety of animal and vegetable products in small amounts, but in large amounts in only a few (see Table A1.7). Foods such as peas, bread, eggs, oranges, potatoes, milk, and cheese supply thiamin in moderate amounts. Cooking easily destroys it, and its other antagonists are caffeine, food-processing methods, oestrogen, and certain drugs. Even exposure to air and water will contribute to its loss.

Table A1.7 Thiamin in foods (DRV 1.5 mg).

Food (portion size)	Thiamin (mg)
Brewer's yeast (10 g)	1.6
Bacon rasher (100 g)	0.8
Pork chop (100 g)	0.5
Bran flakes (50 g)	0.5
Brazil nuts (10 kernels)	0.3
Peanuts (30 kernels)	0.3
Ham (2 slices)	0.3

Riboflavin (vitamin B$_2$)(DRV 1.3 mg men, 1.1 mg women) Riboflavin is present in virtually every living cell, where it helps utilise oxygen and releases energy from carbohydrates and proteins. It is an important component in the pigment of the retina, and is involved in the functioning of the adrenal gland.

The body stores only small amounts of riboflavin, so the DRV of 1.7 mg for men and 1.3 mg for women should be seen as a target to be met every day. It is found in offal, whole-grain foods, and dairy products (see Table A1.8).

Riboflavin is destroyed by light. It is not soluble in water, and so it is not destroyed by cooking, although it is sensitive to heat if sodium bicarbonate is present. Riboflavin is not affected by freezing, but the amount of it in milk is reduced quite considerably by pasteurisation, drying, and evaporation, and milk left in strong light will lose half its riboflavin in a few hours.

Table A1.8 Riboflavin in foods (DRV 1.3 mg men, 1.1 mg women).

Food (portion size)	Riboflavin (mg)
Liver, beef (100 g)	3.0
Kidney (100 g)	2.0
Whole wheat pasta (100 g)	0.7
Brown rice (100 g)	0.6
Cheddar cheese (100 g)	0.5
Yogurt (1 pot, 150 g)	0.4
Cottage cheese, low fat (100 g)	0.2

Niacin (other names: nicotinic acid, vitamin B$_3$)(DRV 18 mg for men and 13 mg for women) Niacin acts as a co-enzyme in the metabolic processes that release the energy of carbohydrates, fats, and proteins in tissue.

Niacin is very stable and can withstand reasonable periods of cooking, heating, and storage (in cans, or by freezing) with little loss. It is water soluble, so some is lost when foods are cooked in water. Very little niacin is stored in the body, so a daily intake is essential, but many common foods, such as fish, meat, and whole-grain foods contain significant amounts (see Table A1.9).

Table A1.9 Niacin in foods (DRV 18 mg men, 13 mg women).

Food (portion size)	Niacin (mg)
Liver, lamb's (100 g)	20
Pork (100 g)	12
Tuna (100 g)	11
Mackerel (100 g)	7.6
Peanuts (30 kernels)	6.5
Sardines, in oil (100 g)	5.4
Bread, wholemeal (2 slices)	4.0
Rice, brown (160 g)	3.0

Pantothenic acid (formerly vitamin B₅) (recommended intake 3–7 mg)

Pantothenic acid plays a vital role in the proper functioning of the adrenal glands. It is essential for the conversion of fat and sugar to energy. It helps in building new tissue, maintaining normal growth, and developing the central nervous system. Pantothenic acid helps wounds heal, fights infection by building antibodies, and prevents fatigue. It is sometimes prescribed as a supplement with certain antibiotics that cause diarrhoea, because it will prevent this side-effect.

Pantothenic acid is found in foods such as offal, mushrooms, and nuts (See Table A1.10). It is water soluble, and is easily destroyed by heat, food-processing techniques, canning, caffeine, sulfa-drugs, sleeping pills, oestrogen, and alcohol.

Table A1.10 Pantothenic acid in foods (recommended intake 3–7 mg).

Food (portion size)	Pantothenic acid (mg)
Peanuts (100 g)	21.5
Liver, lamb's (100 g)	7.8
Kidney, lamb's (100 g)	5.3
Mushrooms (100 g)	2.1
Avocado (200 g)	1.5
Sunflower seeds (100 g)	1.3
Hazelnuts (100 g)	1.1
Muesli (1 bowl, 95 g)	1.1
Egg, medium (60 g)	1.0

Vitamin B₆ See Chapter 10, p. 139.

Biotin (recommended intake 10–200 µg) Biotin is a member of the B vitamin complex, and it plays an important role in metabolising fats, carbohydrates, and proteins. It is absorbed in the early part of the small intestine, and stored in the liver. Beneficial bacteria that occur naturally within the gut manufacture a lot of biotin that our own body can use, as do the so-called probiotic bacteria that are given to colonise the gut and make it healthier. As a consequence, the amount of biotin we excrete in our urine is often many times the amount we take in with out diet.

There are no known toxic effects from an excess of biotin. However, there are two diseases associated with it: one is genetic, and is a rare error in metabolism that can be cured by treating a pregnant woman with massive doses of biotin while the baby is in the womb. The other is a skin disease in infants under six months old, and this responds to dietary supplements.

There is no DRV for biotin, but a daily intake of between 10 and 200 µg should suffice. Foods rich in biotin are cheese, kidney, liver, soya, cauliflower, chocolate, mushrooms, nuts, sardines, salmon, and wheat bran.

Folate See Chapter 10, p. 138.

Vitamin B₁₂ See Chapter 10, p. 141.

Vitamin C See Chapter 10, p. 148.

Vitamin D (chemical name: cholecalciferol) (recommended intake 10 µg)

Vitamin D is often referred to as the sunshine vitamin, because it is formed when sunlight falls on our skin. This is where the body stores it, and it is slowly released from the skin into the blood. Vitamin D promotes the absorption of calcium and phosphate, ensuring the development and health of our bones. Vitamin D deficiency makes the bones soft and pliable, which is called rickets in children and osteomalacia in adults and is very rare today.

Vitamin D is a fat-soluble vitamin found in relatively few foods. It is not lost on cooking, and food containing it can be stored for long periods of time without deterioration. The top ten sources of Vitamin D are oily fish, egg yolk, liver, cream, butter, cheese, and milk, in which it occurs naturally, and breakfast cereals, bread, and margarine, which are fortified with it. Table A1.11 lists typical sources.

Table A1.11 Vitamin D in foods (recommended intake 10 µg).

Food (portion size)	Vitamin D (µg)
Salmon (100 g)	12.5
Sardines in tomato sauce (100 g)	7.5
Tuna (100 g)	5.0
Plain omelette (2 eggs, 100 g)	1.6
Egg, medium (60 g)	1.0
Butter (100 g)	0.8
Liver paté (100 g)	0.6

Vitamin E See Chapter 10, p. 149.

Vitamin K (chemical name: phytomenadione) (recommended intake 70 µg)

Vitamin K is the anti-haemorrhagic vitamin: in other words, it is necessary for blood-clotting, and it prevents excessive bleeding when we cut ourselves.

We can get vitamin K from vegetables in our diet (see Table A1.12), but the bacteria of the small intestine and colon produce almost all that we need, so lack of vitamin K is rare in adults. In new-born babies, however, the gut is sterile, and will remain that way for 3–4 days after birth, until bacteria begin to colonise it. For this reason new-born babies are given an injection of vitamin K to tide them over the risk period.

Vitamin K is not water soluble or damaged by heat, so it is not lost in cooking; but it is lost by exposure to sunlight, and there is some loss with freezing.

Table A1.12 Vitamin K in foods (recommended intake 70 µg).

Food (portion size)	Vitamin K (µg)
Cauliflower (100 g)	3600
Tomatoes (100 g)	400
Spinach (100 g)	400
Runner beans (100 g)	290
Cabbage (100 g)	125
Potatoes (150 g)	120
Brussels sprouts (100 g)	100
Asparagus (100 g)	57
Hard cheese (100 g)	50

Mineral-micronutrients

Copper (DRV 1.2 mg) Copper is an essential nutrient for humans. It is needed for the body to manufacture haemoglobin for the blood, and it is essential for activating many enzyme systems in the metabolic pathways that lead to the production of bone, muscle, and tendon. Occasionally copper poisoning can occur when beverages have been stored in copper containers. Copper is common in a wide range of foods inlcuding liver, nuts, and chocolate (see Table A1.13), and cooking does not interfere with its levels.

Table A1.13 Copper in foods (DRV 1.2 mg).

Food (portion size)	Copper (mg)
Liver (100 g)	12.0
Cashew nuts (100 g)	2.2
Olives (100 g)	1.6
Walnuts (100 g)	1.3
Almonds (100 g)	0.9
Plain (dark) chocolate (100 g)	0.7
Tuna (100 g)	0.6

Iodine (DRV 140 µg) There is only one known role for iodine in the body, and that is in the thyroid gland, where it is needed to make the hormone that governs the amount of heat the body produces by regulating oxidation in cells. This hormone also influences growth. People without enough iodine in their diet suffer from the disfiguring neck condition known as goitre, while those who take in enough iodine, but whose thyroid gland cannot manufacture enough of the thyroid hormone, suffer from lack of energy and continually feel cold. Those with an over-active thyroid gland are hyperactive, restless, and overheated.

To prevent goitre in areas where the soil and the crops grown on it are deficient in iodine, salt is often iodized artificially to provide this element in the diet. Normally most people take in enough iodine from their food, and there are some foods that have high levels, such as dried beans, fish, spinach, and some vegetables (see Table A1.14).

Table A1.14 Iodine in foods (DRV 140 µg).

Food (portion size)	Iodine (µg)
Haddock (100 g)	200
Cod (100 g)	100
Pilchards (100 g)	64
Yoghurt (100 g)	60
Milk, whole, semi-skimmed, or skimmed (half pint)	45
Plaice (100 g)	33
Hard cheese (50 g)	25
Salami (100 g)	15
Corned beef (100 g)	14

Iron (DRV 9 mg men, 15 mg women) There are two forms of iron in food: heme iron, in which the iron atom is part of a large organic molecule, and non-heme iron, which is inorganic. The former is absorbed from foods more efficiently than the latter, and utilising non-heme iron depends on having enough vitamin C in the diet. Ninety per cent of ingested iron is excreted in the faeces, and women lose more, about 14 mg per day, during their menstrual period. Once iron is absorbed into the body it is lost only by the shedding of cells from the gut wall, bladder, respiratory tracts, and skin, and in hair.

Foods with a lot of iron are listed in Table A1.15, but one of the richest sources is cast-iron cookware, which will increase the iron content of food, especially if the food is acidic, whereas boiling food in large amounts of water will cause some of the inorganic iron to be lost.

Table A1.15 Iron in foods (DRV 9 mg men, 15 mg women).

Food (portion size)	Iron (mg)
Branflakes (1 bowl, 45 g)	9
Liver (100 g)	8.8
Beef steak (100 g)	5.4
Corned beef (100 g)	2.9
Haricot beans (100 g)	2.5

Manganese (recommended daily intake 1.4 mg) Manganese is essential for the formation of bone and connective tissue, and for the synthesis of cholesterol. It has a supporting role in the action of insulin and blood clotting, and it is an activator of the enzyme superoxide dismutase, which is part of the body's antioxidant system, and pyruvate carboxylase, which manufactures glucose for the body. Table A1.16 lists foods that are particularly rich in manganese; it is also present in common foods such as baked beans, a can of which contains around 1 mg, and tea, a cup of which contains around 0.3 mg.

Table A1.16 Manganese in foods (recommended daily intake 1.4 mg).

Food (portion size)	Manganese (mg)
Raspberries (100 g)	2.0
Brown rice (100 g)	1.6
Blackberries (100 g)	1.5
Brazil nuts (10 kernels)	1.0
Hazel nuts (30 kernels)	1.0
Grape juice (half pint)	0.9
Pineapple (100 g)	0.8

Selenium   See Chapter 10, p. 143.

Zinc (DRV 10 mg men, 7 mg women)   Zinc is to be found in all parts of the body, and especially in the skin, hair, nails, eyes, and prostate gland. It is an important agent that assists in many metabolic pathways—in this respect, it is the most important metal element after iron. Zinc is needed to keep the immune system healthy; it also stablises the hormone thymosin, which is needed if immature lymphocytes are to develop into mature protective cells. Zinc is plentiful in oysters, and is also found in corn and nuts (see Table A1.17). There is a rapid turnover of zinc in the body, and only a small store to draw upon when insufficient zinc is available from our food. Also, some zinc is rendered inaccessible because of other components in the diet such as phytate (which forms an insoluble salt) or calcium, copper, or cadmium (which are preferentially absorbed) or the chemical EDTA (which is used in canning, and which binds to zinc and carries it from the body).

Table A1.17 Zinc in foods (DRV 10 mg men, 7 mg women).

Food (portion size)	Zinc (mg)
Oysters (12)	78
Popcorn (100 g)	8.3
Sesame seeds (100 g)	7.8
Beef steak (150 g)	7.0
Peanuts (100 g)	4.0
Sardines (100 g)	2.9
Walnuts (100 g)	2.7
Brazil nuts (10 kernels)	1.0

Chromium (recommended daily intake 25 µg) Chromium is important in the metabolism of sugar. It is also an activator for certain enzyme pathways that are involved in the production of energy from carbohydrates, fats, and proteins. It stimulates the digestive enzyme trypsin, and the synthesis of fatty acids and cholesterol in the liver. Chromium is also present in some hormones, and it acts as an assisting agent to some vitamins.

As the body ages, it loses its ability to utilise chromium. Also, its absorption in the gut is opposed by vegetable components such as oxalates, phosphates, and tartrates that are found in rhubarb, spinach, and grapes.

It is suspected that too much high carbohydrate food, such as white sugar and white flour may deplete the body's stores of chromium by overstimulating the release of the mineral from the tissues, followed by its loss in the urine.

The common foods with the highest levels of chromium are eggs, cheese, beef, and potatoes (see Table A1.18).

Table A1.18 Chromium in foods (recommended intake 25 µg).

Food (portion size)	Chromium (µg)
Brewer's yeast (100 g)	118
Cheese (100 g)	51
Liver (100 g)	50
Potatoes (150 g)	36
Beef (100 g)	32
Egg, medium (60 g)	31

Molybdenum (recommended intake 50–400 µg) It is assumed that molybdenum is an essential trace element because it is known to feature in two important metabolic pathways. However, no deficiency syndromes have ever been demonstrated. The enzyme that converts the breakdown products of the cell nucleus to uric acid contains molybdenum (uric acid is responsible for forming the painful crystals in the joints that we experience as gout). Molybdenum is also found in another enzyme, aldehyde hydroxylase.

Molybdenum is easily absorbed from the gut, and is readily excreted in the urine. The total body content of molybdenum is around 5 mg in an adult. Foods rich in molybdenum are listed in Table A1.19.

Table A1.19 Molybdenum in foods (recommended intake 50–400 µg).

Food (portion size)	Molybdenum (µg)
Liver (100 g)	150
Green beans (100 g)	67
Eggs (100 g)	52
Wheat flour (100 g)	49
Chicken (100 g)	42
Spinach (60 g)	25
Cabbage (100 g)	25
Melon (100 g)	17

Much is now known about the chemistry and nutritional make-up of food. However, it is not necessary for the average person to follow the DRVs in the above sections slavishly— we do not have to try to eat the foods that will provide the most of each nutrient, or to buy supplements that will ensure that the minimum requirements are met. Indeed, a gross excess of some vitamins and minerals can cause problems of their own. Our requirements for the various micronutrients can easily be met if we eat a varied diet. The people at risk are those who eat a monotonous diet, choosing to eat the same foods time after time.

Fibre

Fibre is not a nutrient, but it is nevertheless an important component of our diet. Enough fibre should be eaten to ensure one regular bowel movement every day: the recommended daily intake is 30 g. Those who often suffer from constipation would be well advised to increase their intake of fibre, but at the same time they should also drink more—a pint of water with every meal—because fibre absorbs fluid from the intestine as it travels along.

Fibre is not entirely inert. It passes through the small bowel until it reaches the colon, where some of it is broken down by bacteria into short chain fatty acids such as butanoic acid. These fatty acids are needed by the cells lining the colon so that it can function properly; they are also thought to provide protection against colon cancer.

There are two forms of fibre: soluble fibre and insoluble fibre. Soluble fibre is found in fruit, such as bananas, raspberries, olives, apricots, and apples, and in vegetables, such as peas, beans, onions, lentils, and potatoes (especially if the skins are eaten as well as the flesh). Insoluble fibre occurs in bran-based products, such as All-Bran, and in whole wheat products, such as bread, and whole-wheat breakfast cereals such as Weetabix and Shredded Wheat. The fibre in oats is a mixture of soluble and insoluble fibre, and is thought to be particularly beneficial.

Part of dietary fibre is referred to as NSP, short for non-starch polysaccharides, and this includes cellulose, hemicellulose gums, pectins, and lignin. Cellulose and hemicellulose absorb water and are responsible for the smooth functioning of the large bowel, protecting it against diverticulosis, spastic colon, haemorrhoids, and varicose veins. Gums and pectin primarily influence absorption in the stomach, where they delay stomach emptying by coating the lining of the gut, and in the small bowel, where they bind with bile acids. They also inhibit fat absorption, and lower cholesterol levels; but just as important they slow sugar absorption after a meal. This is helpful for people with diabetes, because it reduces the amount of insulin needed at any one time. Lignin binds with bile acids as well as helping essential fats, zinc, and toxins to move along the gut. It is partly for this reason that excessive amounts of fibre in the diet should be avoided: it can interfere with the absorption of some essential minerals by binding to them and carrying them out of the body before they can be utilised.

The NSP component should constitute around 18 g of the total 30 g of fibre in the diet. The remaining 12 g can come from what is referred to as resistant starch, which often forms when food is cooked, and which accounts for much of the fibre in cornflakes, mashed potatoes, spaghetti, white bread, boiled rice, and peas. Resistant starch forms when ordinary

Table A1.20 High fibre foods (recommended daily intake 30 g).

Food (portion size)	Fibre (g)
Baked beans (half a can)	15
All-Bran (50 g)	13
Apricots, dried (100 g)	12
Wholemeal bread (3 slices)	9
Peas (100 g)	8
Prunes, cooked (100 g)	8
Raspberries (100 g)	8
Raisins (100 g)	7
Shredded Wheat (50 g)	7
Sweetcorn (100 g)	6

starch particles stick together so tightly that the digestive enzymes of the stomach and intestines can not break them down. It is only when the starch reaches the colon that the bacteria there can convert some of it into short chain fatty acids, as they do with some of the soluble fibre.

There are lots of foods that provide useful amounts of fibre. All the major manufacturers of breakfast cereals produce one or more varieties that contain either bran or oats. Some fruits and vegetables are particularly rich in fibre, and these are listed in Table A1.20.

Appendix 2: Reference tables

Table A2.1 The tyramine content of foods.

Food	Tyramine content (mg per 100 g)
Drinks	
Beer and ales	0.18–1.12
Wines	0–2.5
Cheeses	
Cheddar	0–150
Camembert	2–200
Emmental	22.5–100
Brie	0–26
Blue or Roquefort	2.7–100
Cottage	0
Edam	30–32
Gruyère	52
Gouda	2–67
Mozzarella	0–41
Boursault	11–111
Povolone	3.8–15
Stilton blue	46–226
Fish	
Tuna	0
Salted dried fish	0–47
Pickled herrings	300
Oyster	unknown*
Perch	unknown*
Nuts	unknown*

Table A2.1 *(continued)*.

Food	Tyramine content (mg per 100 g)
Meat	
Chicken liver	10
Extracts**	9.5–34
Beef liver	27
Sausages	0–124
Pork	unknown*
Fruit and vegetables	
Avocado	2.3
Banana	6.5
Orange	1
Pineapple juice	0.036
Red plum	0.6
Raspberry	1.3–9.3
Prune	0.4
Raisins	unknown*
Sweet potato	unknown*
Radish	unknown
Spinach	unknown*
Tomato	unknown*
Potato	unknown*
Green peas	unknown*
Other foods	
Soya sauce	1–7.6
Yeast extracts	0–226
Eggs	unknown*
Cows milk	unknown*

*Tyramine is present, but the quantity is unknown. However, if these foods start to go off then the level of tyramine can go up rapidly.
**Meat extracts which are added as constituents in manufactured food or are provided as cooking aids such as Bovril, gravy cubes etc.

The data in Table A2.2, and in Tables 5.1 and 5.2, come from a paper published in 1985 in the *Journal of the American Dietetic Association* by Anne Swain and her colleagues. They extracted the salicylic acid from 333 foods and drinks, and employed a sensitive analytical technique, high-performance liquid chromatography, to measure the amount of the acid. Their results showed that most foods contain salicylate, but the amounts vary widely. For example, in vegetables the amount of salicylate can be as low as zero (in celery) and as high as 6 mg per 100 g (in gherkins). The typical portion sizes are taken from *Nutrient Content of Food Portions* by Jill Davies and John Dickerson (Royal Society of Chemistry, London, 1991).

Table A2.2 The salicylate content of foods.

Food	Salicylate content (mg per 100 g)	Typical portion	Salicylate intake (mg)
Fruits			
Apple, Golden Delicious	0.08	1 (120 g)	0.01
Apple, Granny Smith	0.59	1 (120 g)	0.71
Avocado	0.60	half (130 g)	0.78
Cantaloupe melon	1.50	half (360 g)	4.68
Cherries	0.85	12 (100 g)	0.85
Grapes	0.94	cluster (140 g)	1.32
Currants	5.80	2 handfuls (35 g)	2.03
Raisins	6.62	2 handfuls (30 g)	2.32
Grapefruit	0.68	6 segments (120 g)	0.82
Mango	0.11	1 (315 g)	0.35
Orange	2.39	1 (245 g)	5.86
Peach	0.58	1 (125 g)	0.73
Pear	0.27	1 (150 g)	0.41
Pineapple	2.10	1 slice (125 g)	2.63
Raspberries	5.14	15 (70 g)	3.60
Strawberries	1.6	1 serving (100 g)	1.60
Watermelon	0.48	1 slice (320 g)	2.46
Vegetables			
Asparagus	0.14	4 spears (120 g)	0.17
Broad beans	0.73	1 serving (75 g)	0.55
French beans	0.11	1 serving (105 g)	0.12
Broccoli	0.65	1 serving (95 g)	0.62
Brussels sprouts	0.07	1 serving (115 g)	0.08
Carrot	0.23	1 serving (65 g)	0.15
Cauliflower	0.16	1 serving (100 g)	0.16
Leek	0.08	1 serving (125 g)	0.10
Marrow/Squash	0.17	1 serving (90 g)	0.15
Mushroom	0.24	1 serving (55 g)	0.13
Onion	0.16	1 serving (40 g)	0.06
Parsnip	0.45	1 serving (110 g)	0.50
Peas	0.04	1 serving (75 g)	0.03
Potato, whole	0.12	1 serving (140 g)	0.17
Spinach	0.58	1 serving, (130 g)	0.75
Sweet corn, fresh	0.13	1 cob (70 g)	0.09
Sweet corn, canned	0.26	1 serving (70 g)	0.18
Turnip	0.16	1 serving (140 g)	0.22
Courgette/Zucchini	1.04	1 serving (140 g)	1.46
Salads			
Beetroot, boiled	0.18	1 serving (40 g)	0.07
Chicory	1.02	1 serving (45 g)	0.46
Cucumber	0.78	1 serving (30 g)	0.23
Gherkin	0.78	1 (20 g)	0.16

Table A2.2 *(continued).*

Food	Salicylate content (mg per 100 g)	Typical portion	Salicylate intake (mg)
Olive, black (canned)	0.34	9 (35 g)	0.12
Olive, green (canned)	1.29	9 (35 g)	0.45
Red pepper	1.20	1 serving (45 g)	0.54
Sesame seeds	0.23	sprinkling (25 g)	0.04
Tomato	0.13	2 (150 g)	0.20
Nuts			
Almonds	3.0	20 kernels (20 g)	0.60
Brazil nuts	0.46	9 kernels (30 g)	0.14
Cashew nuts	0.07	20 kernels (40 g)	0.03
Coconut, desiccated	0.26	1 serving (50 g)	0.13
Peanuts	1.12	32 (30 g)	0.34
Walnuts	0.30	9 halves (25 g)	0.08
Drinks			
Orange juice	0.18	1 glass (200 ml)	0.36
Tomato juice	0.12	1 glass (200 ml)	0.24
Coca-Cola	0.25	1 glass (200 ml)	0.50
Coffee*			
fresh beans	0.45	1 cup	0.45
Maxwell House	0.84	1 cup	0.84
Nescafé	0.59	1 cup	0.55
Tea**			
Tetley	5.57	1 cup	5.57
Earl Grey	3.00	1 cup	3.00
Darjeeling	4.24	1 cup	4.24
*Alcoholic drinks***			
Beer	*c.* 0.3	1 glass (500 ml)	*c.* 1.5
Cider	*c.* 0.2	1 glass (500 ml)	*c.* 1.0
Benedictine liqueur	9.04	1 glass (25 ml)	2.26
Cointreau	0.66	1 glass (25 ml)	0.17
Port	2	1 glass (50 ml)	*c.* 1
Sherry	0.5	1 glass (50 ml)	*c.* 0.25
Brandy	*c.* 0.4	1 glass (25 ml)	*c.* 0.1
Wine	0.8	1 glass (125 ml)	*c.* 1
Other foods			
Honey	2.5–11.24	1 teaspoon (7 g)	0.18–0.79
Golden syrup	0.10	1 teaspoon (7 g)	0.01
Licorice	9.78	as allsorts (25 g)	2.44
Peppermint sweets	0.77–7.58	1 tube (30 g)	0.23–2.77
Peanut butter	0.23	1 spreading (7 g)	0.02
Tomato ketchup	2.48	1 serving (20 g)	0.05
Tomato soup, Heinz	0.54	1 bowl (145 ml)	0.78
Marmite (yeast extract)	0.71	1 spreading (4 g)	0.03
Worcester sauce	64.3	1 teaspoon (7 g)	4.50

*Instant coffee: 2 g powder in 100 ml water.

**Tea: two tea bags in 100 ml water.

***Varies according to brewery, orchard, and vineyard.

Further reading

A. Albert, *Xenobiosis, Food, Drugs and Poisons in the Human Body*, Chapman & Hall, London, 1987.

R. Bates (ed.), *What Risk?* Butterworth Heinemann for the European Science and Environment Forum, Oxford, 1997.

S. H.-D. Belitz and W. Grosch, *Food Chemistry*, Springer Verlag, Berlin, 1987.

E. Bender, *Health or Hoax?* Sphere Books Ltd, London, 1986.

S. Bingham, *The Everyman Companion to Food and Nutrition*, J.M. Dent & Sons Ltd, London, 1987.

S. Braun, *Buzz*, Oxford University Press, New York, 1996.

J. Brostoff and L. Gamlin, *The Complete Guide to Food Allergy and Intolerance*, Bloomsbury London, 1989.

G. F. Combs Jr, and S. B. Combs, *The Role of Selenium in Nutrition*, Academic Press, Orlando, 1987.

T. P. Coultate, *Food, the Chemistry of its Components*, 3rd edition, Royal Society of Chemistry, London, 1995.

S. D. Coe and M. D. Coe, *The True History of Chocolate*, Thames and Hudson, London, 1996.

A. P. Cox and P. Brusseau, *Secret Ingredients*, Bantam Books, London, 1997.

T. J. David, *Food and Food Additive Sensitivity in Childhood*, Blackwell Scientific, Oxford, 1991.

R. L. Duyff, *Complete Food & Nutrition Guide*, American Dietetic Association, Chronimed Publishing, Minneapolis, 1996.

J. Davies and J. Dickerson, *Nutrient Content of Food Portions*, Royal Society of Chemistry, London, 1991.

A. H. Ensminger, *The Concise Encyclopedia of Foods and Nutrition*, CRC Press, Boca Raton, USA, 1995.

K. T. H. Farrer, *A Guide to Food Additives and Contaminants*, Parthenon Publishing Group, Carnforth, 1987.

M. Hanssen, *E for Additives*, Thorsons, Wellingborough, Northampton, 1994.

M. Henderson (ed.), *Living with Risk,* The British Medical Association Guide, John Wiley & Sons, Chichester, 1987.

H. Hobhouse, *Seeds of Change: Five Plants that Transformed Mankind,* Sidgwick & Jackson, London, 1985.

J. T. Hughes, *Aluminium and Your Health,* Rimes House, Cirencester, UK, 1992.

M. H. Jackson, G. P. Morris, P. G. Smith and J. F. Crawford, *Environmental Health,* Butterworth-Heinemann, London, 1989.

F. Katch and W. McArdie, *Introduction to Nutrition, Exercise and Health,* Lea & Febigier, Philadelphia, 1993.

R. J. Kutsky, *Handbook of Vitamins, Minerals and Hormones,* 2nd edition, Van Nostrand Reinhold, New York, 1981.

J. Lenihan, *The Crumbs of Creation,* Adam Hilger, Bristol, 1988.

T. D. Luckey and B. Venugopal, *Metal Toxicity in Mammals,* Plenum Press, New York, 1977.

J. Mann, *Murder, Magic and Medicine,* Oxford University Press, Oxford, 1994.

P. Mason, *Handbook of Dietary Supplements,* Blackwell Science, Oxford, 1995.

A. McWhirter and L. Clasen (eds), *Food That Harm and Foods That Heal,* Reader's Digest, London, 1996.

W. Mertz (ed), *Trace Elements in Human and Animal Nutrition,* Academic Press, San Diego, 1987.

L. Mervyn, *Vitamins and Minerals,* Thorsons, Wellingborough, Northampton, 1989.

D. Metcalfe, H. Simpson and R. Simon, *Food Allergy,* Blackwell Scientific, Oxford, 1991.

A. Ottoboni, *The Dose Makes the Poison,* 2nd edition, Van Nostrand Reinhold, New York, 1991.

A. A. Paul and D. A. T. Southgate, *McCance and Widdowson's The Composition of Foods,* 4th edition, HMSO, London, 1988.

J. Postgate, *Microbes and Man,* 3rd edition, Penguin Books, London, 1992.

C. A. Rinzler, *Food Facts and What They Mean,* Bloomsbury, London, 1987.

J. V. Rodricks, *Calculated Risks: Understanding the Toxicity and Health Risks of Chemicals in Our Environment,* Cambridge University Press, Cambridge, 1992.

B. Saunders, *Understanding Additives,* UK Consumers' Association, Hodder & Stoughton, London, 1988.

J. A. Timbrell, *Introduction to Toxicology,* Taylor & Francis, London, 1989.

UK Department of Health, *Dietary Reference Values for Food Energy and Nutrients for the United Kingdom,* Report of the Panel on Dietary Reference Values of the Committee on Medical Aspects of Food Policy, Report No. 41, HMSO, London, 1991.

US Food and Drug Administration, *Food Borne Pathogenic Microorganisms and Natural Toxins Report,* Washington, 1992.

J. G. Vaughan and C. A. Geissler, *The New Oxford Book of Food Plants,* Oxford University Press, Oxford, 1997.

H. Watson (ed), *Natural Toxicants in Food,* VCH-Ellis Horwood, Chichester, 1987.

E. M. Whelan, *Toxic Terror,* Prometheus Books, Buffalo, 1993.

Glossary

Adenosine This compound is one of the nucleosides that make up the genetic code, and it consists of an organic base, a sugar, and a phosphate group.

Adrenal glands These glands are situated on top of the, kidneys, and consist of two parts: the cortex (in the centre), and the medulla (the outer part). The cortex produces corticosteroids, which are essential hormones controlling a variety of bodily functions, such as producing the sex hormones and the precursors of sex hormones. The medulla produces adrenalin and noradrenalin, the so-called 'fight or flight' hormones.

Aflatoxin This is a toxin produced by moulds and associated with foods as they degrade. Some foods have a naturally high content of aflatoxin. The European Union sets a limit for animal feedstuffs at 20–50 μg per kg.

Aldehydes These are chemicals characterised by having molecules that have as part of their make-up a carbon atom to which is attached a hydrogen atom and an oxygen atom, the latter being held to the carbon by a double bond. Aldehydes are represented by the general fomula R-CHO where R is an organic group.

Amino acids These compounds are the basic units from which protein is assembled. They are either produced in the body as required, or absorbed from the digestion of food proteins. Some are termed 'essential' amino acids, which indicates that they must be obtained by the latter route, since they can not be manufactured in the body.

Amphetamines These drugs indirectly stimulate the pathways governed by adrenalin and noradrenalin, and consequently they increase arousal, decrease appetite, and accelerate many bodily functions.

Anaphylactic shock   is an extremely rapid reaction, usually allergy-induced but occasionally chemically induced, that leads to total functional collapse. It is often fatal because it needs immediate treatment which may not be available. People at risk of this, such as those allergic to peanuts, usually need to carry the antidotes adrenalin and antihistamine with them at all times.

Antibodies These are complex proteins called gamma-globulins that protect us from a range of hostile things inlcuding bacteria, viruses, and poisons. One antibody, IgE, is manufactured by allergic individuals in response to what should be harmless compounds, and this causes their symptoms to develop when they are in contact with the offending materials.

Anti-haemorrhagic agents   are cells, compounds, and systems in the body that prevent bleeding or block it after it has started. Haemophiliacs lack these agents, and they will bleed excessively after damage, or even spontaneously.

Arterial system   This system consists of the heart, the large blood vessels leaving it, the smaller blood vessels distributing the oxygenated blood to the organs, and the capillaries, which are the smallest blood vessels.

Aspirin   See salicylic acid.

Bronchial asthma   is a disease in which the lungs, or, more precisely the bronchi (the tubes), either go into spasm or produce too much mucous, or both. This term was once more common because it was used to distinguish this type of asthma from cardiac asthma, in which the heart malfunctions.

Buffers   These are chemicals that prevent too great a shift from acidic to alkali conditions, or vice versa, when a chemical change is occurring.

Chloracne   Acne-like pimples on the skin which generally occur on the hands and face, and are caused by exposure to chlorinated hydrocarbons.

Chloramphenicol   This antibiotic is now rarely prescribed to be taken orally because of its toxicity, but it is commonly used in preparations such as eye-drops.

Cholesterol   This is a steroid with important and essential functions in the body. It is the precursor to many hormones. Most cholesterol in the body is manufactured by the liver but some is absorbed from the diet, and certain foods contain a lot. It has been implicated in heart disease and is now recognised as a risk factor if high levels are present in the blood.

Cholinesterase   Acetylcholine is a neurotransmitter responsible for the activation of nerves that are vital to the function of several organs, including the gut and brain. Once activation has occurred, the acetylcholine needs to be eliminated by the enzyme cholinesterase.

Colorectal   refers to the large intestine from its beginning, the caecum, to its end, the rectum.

Curare-like   Drugs are described as curare-like when they produce paralysis. They are used mainly in anaesthesia to relax organs during operations, particularly those of the gut.

Cyclooxygenase   enzymes assist in the manufacture of prostaglandins, a group of chemicals that are active in the reproductive system. Prostaglandins also govern the secretory activity of organs such as the stomach, and control blood pressure and inflammatory responses.

Detoxifying enzymes   are used to disable potentially toxic molecules so that they may be excreted from the body.

Dexfenfluramine   is a drug used in dieting.

Diazepam   is a minor tranquilliser that is used to control panic attacks, reduce anxiety, and relax muscles. Its trade name is Valium.

Diverticulosis   This is a disease of the large intestine that develops usually in the second half of life. It is caused by pressure on the intestine, leading to the development of protruding pouches on the intestine wall.

Double-blind test   This is a technique used for evaluating drugs and other test materials in clinical trials. It entails both the observer and the patient being unaware of whether the test material, or an inactive placebo, is being used.

Enzymes   These are small peptides (proteins) designed to perform specific chemical changes. Most metabolic pathways would be too slow to react without the help of enzyme catalysts to speed them up.

Epidemiology   This is the science of studying the effects of disease, its prevention and its treatment in large populations of patients to determine what factors are statistically significant.

Free radicals   These are molecules with an active electron, and as such they tend to be extremely reactive, attacking almost anything within range. Because of the damage they are potentially capable of causing, such as to a cell's DNA, the body needs a supply of antioxidants that can mop up free radicals as soon as they are formed.

Glycogen   is the main energy store in the body. Glucose is converted to glycogen for storage when it is in excess, and the glycogen is broken down into glucose when this is short supply. In this way, blood glucose levels remain stable.

Gram-negative bacteria   A method of identifying bacteria is to stain them with dye, called Gram stain, and then look at them under the microscope. Those taking up the dye are Gram-positive, those unstained are Gram-negative.

Haemoglobin   The complex iron-containing molecule in the red blood cells that enables oxygen to be carried around the body to the tissues.

Haemorrhoids   Commonly known as 'piles', these are varicose veins situated at the anus, and they are the result of pressure on the veins producing a bulge similar to those seen on the inner tube of tyres.

Host reaction   When an organism is invaded by hostile agents—viruses, bacteria, fungi, poisons—a number of defence systems are activated to fight them, and this is known as the host reaction.

Hydrocortisone   This is the hormone that is released by the adrenal cortex. It controls a wide range of activities in the body.

Hypokalaemia   is a low level of blood potassium.

Hypothalamus   This part of the brain regulates many functions. At its base is the pituitary gland, which releases hormones controlling sexual function, the adrenal cortex and thyroid glands, growth, lactation, and several other essential actions.

Insulin   This hormone is secreted by the pancreas, and controls the amount of glucose in the blood. Insulin deficiency leads to diabetes mellitus; on rare occasions there can be an excess of insulin due to a pancreatic tumour.

Ketones   These are chemicals characterised by a group of three linked carbon atoms with an oxygen atom attached to the middle carbon by a double bond. Ketones are represented by the general formula $R_1R_2C{=}O$ where R_1 and R_2 are organic groups.

Microorganisms   This is the generic term for microscopic organisms: it embraces viruses, bacteria, yeasts, fungi, and single-cell amoeba-like parasites.

Migraine   This distinct type of headache is caused by the blood vessels in the head first contracting, then dilating. The consequences are visual flashes of colour and a sensitivity to noise, followed by a thumping headache. A migraine is usually on one side of the head, and can sometimes be so severe as to cause paralysis. This is then often followed by nausea or vomiting, which may continue for several hours. (There are many examples of migraines that do not fit these patterns.)

Monoamine oxidase inhibitor (MAOI)   Monoamine oxidase is the enzyme that breaks down histamine and some of the other biogenic amines. If it is blocked by an inhibitor, there will be an increase in the level amines in the body. The monoamine oxidase inhibitors have a beneficial effect in cases of depression, and they have been prescribed for more than thirty years.

Myelin sheath   This surrounds and protects nerves.

Neurotransmitter   Nerves are triggered by molecules called neurotransmitters. There are over forty varieties in the body, all performing different functions.

Osmotic pressure   When two solutions containing dissolved salts or other chemicals are separated by a semi-permeable membrane, a pressure difference develops towards the side with the higher concentration, and this enables movement of water across the membrane. This pressure is referred to as osmotic pressure.

Osteomalacia   is a state of deficiency of minerals, primarily calcium and phosphorus, in bone.

Oxidising   is the addition of an oxygen atom to a molecule. This is one of the most important detoxifying mechanisms in the body, but it is also one of the processes that occur when food goes off.

Palpitations   This is an awareness of the heartbeat and is extremely common, more so in women, coffee drinkers, and smokers. Palpitations can be regular or irregular, acute or sometimes chronic, and are usually of no consequence. Grossly irregular or persistent palpitations need further investigation, and medical help should be sought.

Pancreas   This organ is situated in the upper abdomen close to the stomach and duodenum. A duct connects the pancreas to the duodenum, enabling the digestive juices it produces to be released into the gut when the stomach empties. Within the pancreas there are 'islands' that manufacture and release insulin directly into the blood stream.

Paraldehyde   This drug was used in epilepsy to abort a fit, and for a variety of conditions where fits might be a problem. Not much used nowadays, it has been superseded by more sophisticated drugs.

Parasthesae   These are sensations caused by nerve stimulation, and are commonly referred to as pins and needles.

Parkinson's disease   This is a disorder of co-ordination, and it is usually due to a deterioration of the supply of blood to a group of structures known as the basal ganglia in the brain. The result is a tremor, a strange rigidity in the limbs called 'cogwheel', and 'mask-like' facial features. The condition is progressive but often responds well to treatment.

Phospholipids   These are body chemicals that are part of cell membranes. Choline and inositide phospholipids are found throughout the body, and serine phospholipid is concentrated in the brain.

Phytic acid   This is a phosphorus-containing derivative of inositol, and is found in cereals, nuts, and grains. It naturally binds to certain minerals such as zinc, iron, and calcium, and can prevent these from being absorbed from the gut.

Placenta   This organ controls the nutrition, oxygenation, and removal of waste for the fetus while in the womb. It also allows defensive antibodies to cross from the mother to protect the baby.

Plasma   Blood consists of white cells, red cells, and platelets suspended in a complex of dissolved chemicals called plasma.

Platelets   These are the smallest particles in the blood, and they serve several vital functions: they stop bleeding by clumping, they set up inflammatory responses, and they release chemicals when activated.

Probiotics   are the useful bacteria that live in the gut and provide 25% of the body's energy needs. They help shift important minerals and vitamins across the gut wall, and help the gut wall to stay healthy.

Prostaglandins   These are a group of compounds that are needed for the manufacture of steroids, corticosteroids, and sex hormones. They control such vital functions as ovulation, birth, gastric secretion, clotting, fever, inflammation, and pain.

Prothrombin   is an important protein that is an integral part of the clotting mechanism.

Psychosis   A psychosis is a serious psychiatric disorder that is not easily cured, as opposed to 'neurosis', which embraces the majority of common psychiatric disturbances including anxiety, depression, and panic attacks. Schizophrenia is a psychosis.

Psychosomatic   means a mental condition rather than an organic disorder, often now called somatisation, in which the body develops symptoms without an underlying physical cause.

Rapid eye movement   This is a stage of sleep that usually follows the deepest level. It is thought to be the time during which the day's information is catalogued and sorted in the brain. It is characterised by the flickering of the eyelids and twitching of the muscles.

Receptors   are the sites that trigger the various functions of the body, and they are activated by specific molecules.

Respiratory alkalosis   An increase in breathing rate, known as hyperventilation, will wash out carbon dioxide from the blood, which becomes alkaline as this acidic gas is removed. This alkaline state is respiratory alkalosis. The reverse process will cause the acidity of the blood to rise, and produce respiratory acidosis.

Reye's syndrome   This rare syndrome has a relatively high incidence in children under twelve years old who are given medications containing aspirin. Because of the risk of Reye's syndrome, aspirin is now not recommended for children.

Salicylic acid and salicylate   This acid has the chemical formula $C_6H_4(OH)(CO_2H)$, and is a derivative of phenol with a carboxylic acid group (CO_2H) attached to the benzene ring and adjacent to the OH group. Salicylates are derivatives of this acid, in which the H of the carboxylic acid has been replaced. Aspirin is acetyl salicylic acid, in which the H of the OH group has been replaced by an acetyl group ($COCH_3$).

Salivary fluid   Saliva is produced from three sets of glands in the region of the mouth—the parotids, submandibular, and sublingual glands—which are stimulated even by the sight of food. Saliva contains the enzyme amylase, which breaks down complex carbohydrates, and starts the first stage of digestion as the food is chewed.

Salmonella   are bacteria that cause the commonest form of food-borne infection. They are rarely fatal and are killed by adequate cooking.

Schizophrenia   This psychiatric disorder is characterised by irrational thoughts, and can take a wide variety of forms. It responds well to treatment.

Spastic colon   This disorder of the large bowel is characterised by irregular muscular contractions. It is now more commonly known as irritable bowel syndrome.

Syndrome   is a condition identified by a collection of symptoms.

Thyroid gland   This gland, which is situated in the neck, produces the hormone thyroxine that determines the body's rate of metabolism. Too much thyroxine leads to weight loss, a rapid pulse, and a sensation of heat (thyrotoxic), while too little causes weight increase, slowness, and a feeling of cold (myxoedema).

Toxins   are compounds produced by plants, animals, and microbes that cause adverse effects when ingested.

Trypsin   is an enzyme in the gastric and gut juices that breaks down complex proteins.

Ureters   are the tubes that connect the kidneys to the bladder.

Urticaria   is a skin condition characterised by weals and flares on the skin that are extremely irritating. It is commonly known as hives.

Varicose veins   form in the legs and elsewhere when the valves that control the flow of blood are malfunctioning, causing a back-pressure of blood. This pressure produces small grape-like swellings in the veins.

Index